REIKI PRACTITIONER

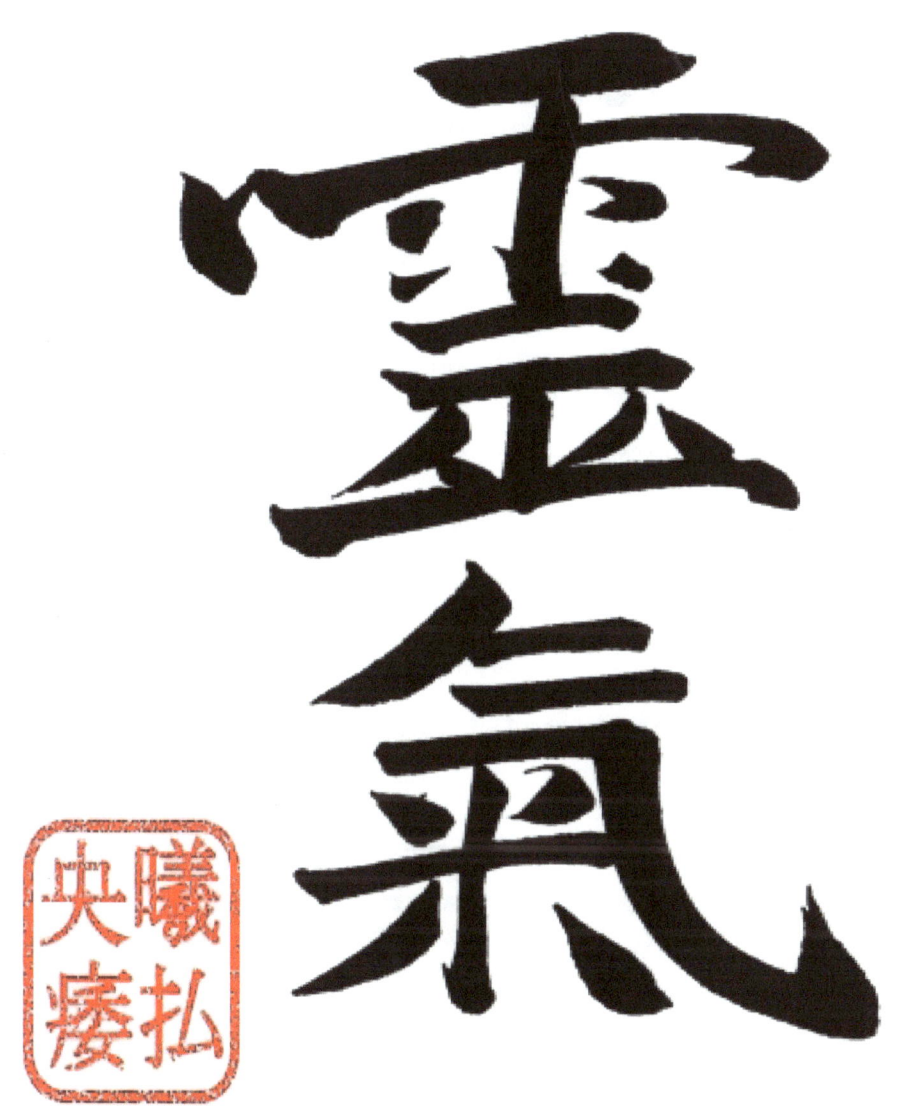

ESSENTIAL BOOK IN THE
PRACTICAL HEALING ROOM

Reiki- 1

<u>Instructed by:</u>

M. & E. Moghazy

Grand Master Teachers

This training has been designed

for whom wants to become

A Certified Reiki Natural Healing Practitioner.

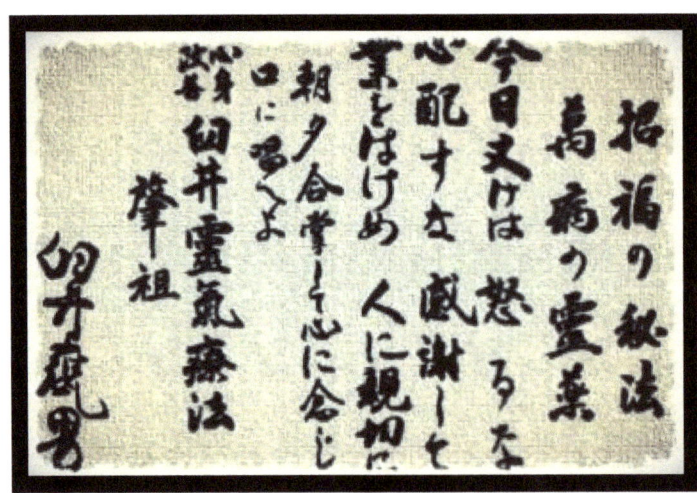

Acknowledgments and Thanks

I am extremely grateful to who have been such profoundly positive influence on my life and my spiritual path and to those who have informed and inspired me with their teaching and work.

For My Wife, My Family, those who in form of divine guidance, Teachers, Masters, Angels who are always with me, who always love, help encourage and reassure me, who give me insight, understanding and healing, I thank you and I thank God.

Disclaimer

Healing and medicine are two very different disciplines, and the law requires the following disclaimer: The information in this Manual is not Medicine but Healing, and does not constitute medical advice. In case of serious illness consult your practitioner of choice.

Curriculum Content

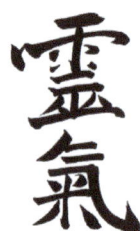

Section 1: Chapter 1- Reiki Level I

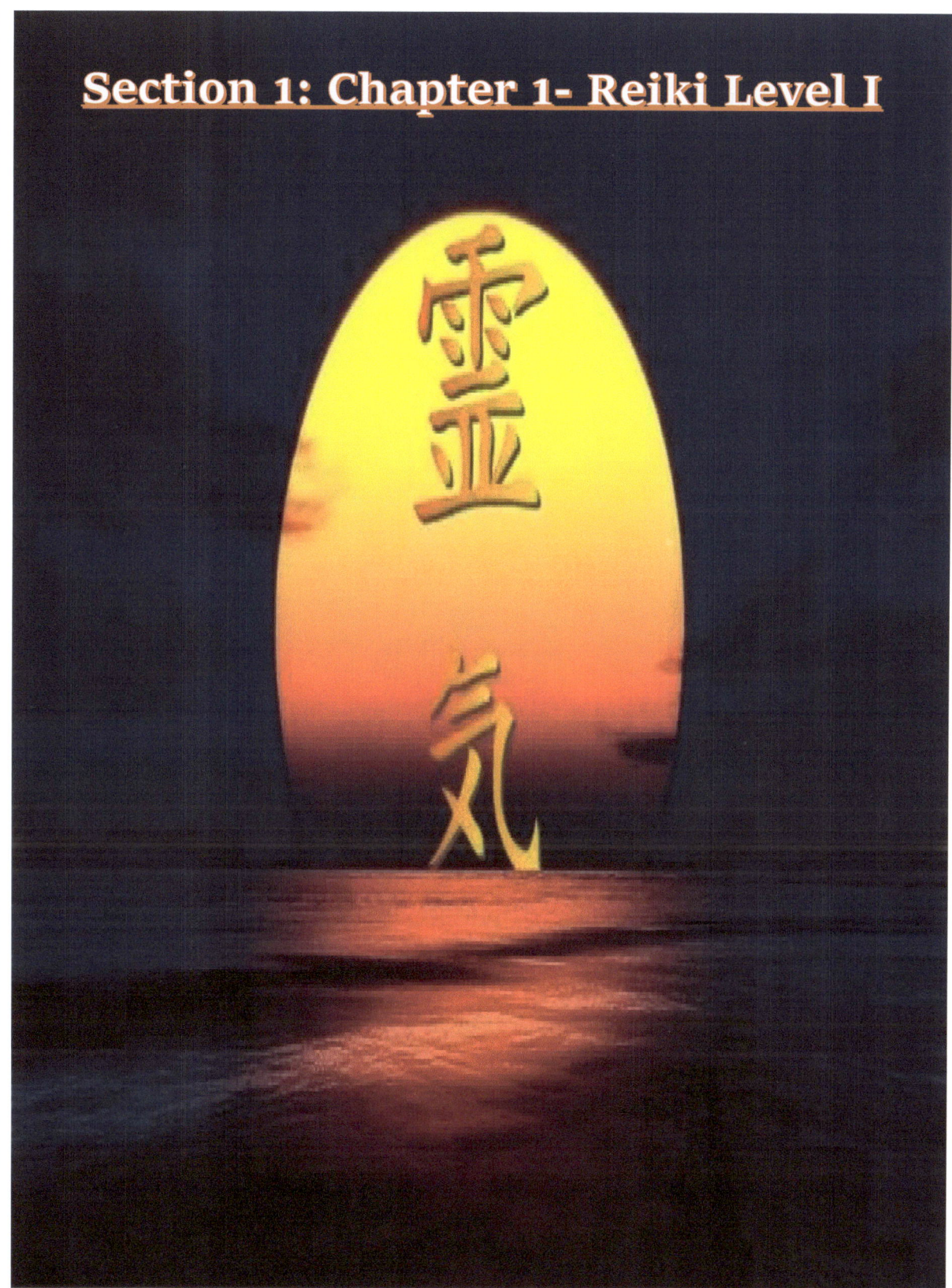

Course Description:

Learning Reiki, A Universal Natural Energy Healing Method that has been used successfully all over the world for millions of years to heal emotional, physical and energetic imbalances. In this course you will learn how to perform Reiki on yourself and others.

This course is designed for the Healthcare Professional to help themselves and their patients reduce fatigue, empower patient centered healing and rejuvenate the spirit of participating professionals. This is done by offering integrative skills that can be offered in the work place and at the patient's bedside. These techniques may also be used by the professional in their private lives to enhance personal well-being.

You will receive this comprehensive manual as well as your Professional Certificate as a Qualified Reiki Practitioner. You will receive the attunement for Reiki level I from Ezzat Your Master Teacher, who has been in the healthcare industry nearly 16 years. He offers international experience, traveling all over the world and collecting the most tangible knowledge in the Reiki Energy Natural Healing techniques. He is able to give the Healthcare Professionals the power over their daily practice. Helping their patients with accelerating the healing process.

The Levels of Reiki

Reiki training has three levels.

A Certified Reiki Practitioner Level I

- **Level 1** provides a foundation of knowledge about the practice, its origins, the nature of Reiki energy, and how it can promote healing.

A Certified Reiki Therapist Level II

- **Level 2** provides instruction on using Reiki for distance healing, energy exercises to strengthen Reiki practice, and use of Reiki-specific symbols in healing.

A Certified Reiki Master Teacher Level III

- **Level 3** prepares the practitioner to use additional Reiki tools to facilitate healing and teach Reiki to others.

What are the requirements?

There are no course requirements. This training has been designed for the Healthcare Professional who wants to become highly qualified as "A certified Reiki Practitioner"

What is the target audience?

This Reiki Certificate training course provides education of holistic self-healing techniques and training for health care professionals working in any clinical or nonclinical setting facilities including but not limited to hospitals, maternity, mental health, rehabilitation, managed care, home-bound or disabled, assisted living, palliative, and hospice.

What am I going to get from this course?

Why take this course?

The Course Outcome / Benefits:

#1 Over 8.5 hours of content! You will get a direct contact with the Grand Master Teacher, who has taught this course all over the world, between UK, EUROPE, SOUTH AFRICA, DUBAI, USA and more.

#2 Reiki as a healing and personal growth system.

#3 The major benefits of the Reiki course for the Healthcare Professionals is the powerful relaxation and healing modality that can be used both for self-care and in assisting health care providers with treatment outcomes for pain management and other chronic diseases.

#4 In this course nurses in any clinical or non-clinical setting as well as in private practice will learn what Reiki is: how reiki works; uses of reiki, an introduction to the human energy system; comprehensive hand positions for working with patients, self-care and much more.

#5 You will learn in this comprehensive Reiki course particularly designed for Healthcare providers that Reiki is a non-invasive, natural system of healing thus provides stress-relief, pain management, deep calming relaxation and balance without medication or traditional medical applications.

#6 The healing knowledge in this course will help you, your family, your patients to live better and happier.

#7 This Reiki course is a natural extension of nursing's knowledge and skills, and can have a powerful impact on today's health care system.

#8 You will learn and experience the benefits of regular meditation and relaxation techniques.

#9 Chakra locations and effects of imbalance's.

Chapter 2: Introduction to Reiki

Reiki is a hands on form of healing practice like all other healthcare professions, pronounced (RAY-KEY), and it has two components; Rei – Means Universal and Ki – means Life force.

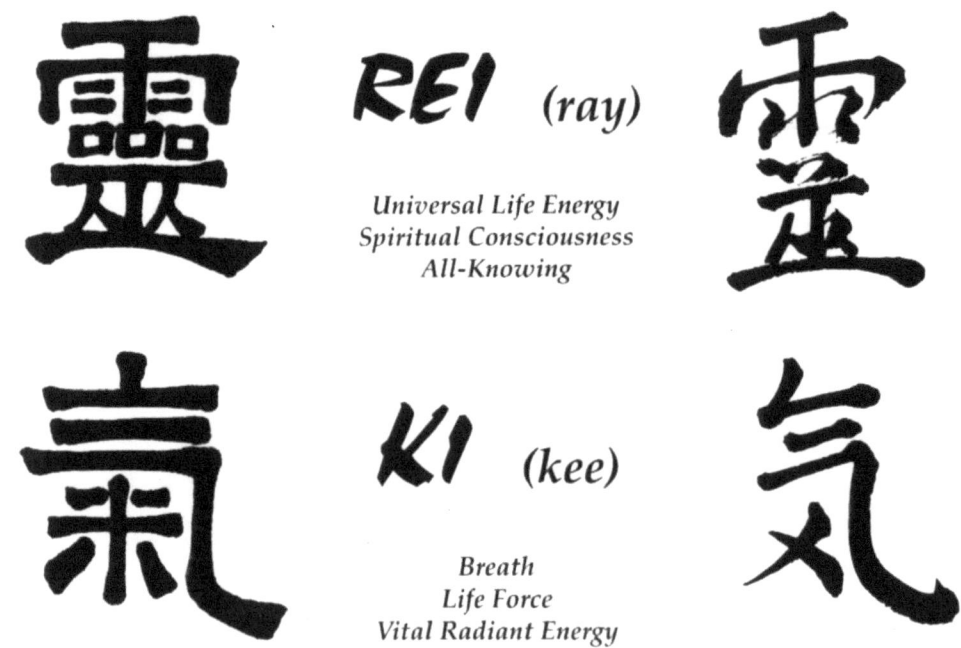

Reiki is a wonderful gift that can help you to change your life for the better. By deciding to become a Reiki practitioner and receiving the Reiki First Degree attunement you become directly connected to a powerful, divine healing energy source. Reiki is practiced all over the world by thousands, if not millions of Healthcare professionals and it is an absolutely safe and very powerful way of channeling healing energy.

In The Reiki first degree the student will receive what we call it the "attunement" and the attunements means creates a channel for divine love and healing so that the initiate can channel pure healing energy to their selves, other people and things.

I choose to teach Reiki Certifications for the Healthcare Professionals primarily due to my background as a Physical Therapist of 16 years. Which opened the avenue to become and a Certified Reiki Practitioner and Master teacher. I originally was taught back in 1999. My Master Teacher was very traditional and did not believe in manuals or certification paper. It was only later in 2010 that I was recertified to possess the actual certificate, which is sought over these days for recognition. After becoming a Reiki Master, I was able to experience the most advanced healing modalities and places throughout the USA, UK, Europe, South Africa, Dubai, Japan and experienced healing first hand, all over the world. Through my travels around the world, I have healed and been healed, I have been a teacher and been taught.

Reiki is a powerful natural healing method, I want to continue sharing my very humble 16 years of healing and Teaching experience with my colleagues in the healthcare industry. I want to teach the old traditions along with the newer modern practices of Reiki for professionals such as yourself. In addition, I want to share with you, as healthcare professional how to make another person's life better. During this Reiki course which is a natural extension to your knowledge and skill set as a health care professional, you can help to make a powerful improvement towards today's health care system.

Chapter 3: How Reiki Works?

We are alive thanks to a life force, which flows through us and from us. This life force flows within the physical body through pathways called Chakras and Meridians. It also flows around us in a field of energy called the Aura. Life force nourishes the organs and the cells of the body, supporting them in their vital functions. When this flow of life force is disrupted, it disturbs the functions in one or more of the organs and tissues of the physical body.

The life force is responsive to thoughts and feelings. It becomes disrupted when we accept, either consciously or unconsciously, negative thoughts or feelings about ourselves or others. Negative thoughts and feelings are not something that disappears into thin air; rather they attach themselves to the energy field and cause blockages. According to Quantum Physics, thoughts affect the arrangement of the atoms that make up the physical bodies. Negative thoughts can, if allowed, diminish the vital functions of the organs of the physical body.

Reiki heals by flowing through the affected parts of the energy field and charging them with positive energy. It raises the vibrations of the energy field in and around the physical body where negative thoughts and feelings are attached. This causes the negative energy to break apart. In so doing, Reiki clears, straightens, heals and balances the energy pathways, thus allowing the life force to flow in a healthy and natural way.

While giving a Reiki treatment, the brain wave patterns of the practitioner and the receiver become synchronized in the alpha state, characteristic of deep relaxation and meditation, and pulsing in unison with the universe magnetic field. During these moments, the bio-magnetic field of the practitioners' hands is at least 1000 times greater than normal.

The linking of energy fields allows the practitioner to draw on the universal energy field. The healer is only a channel for this gentle and loving energy. The healer or the healer's mind, cannot guide it, therefore it cannot be misused.

About Reiki Healing in the Healthcare Industry

Reiki (pronounced ray-key) healing is a practice that is probably thousands of years old. It is thought to have first been used by Tibetan monks but was rediscovered in the late 1800's by Dr. Mikao Usui, a Japanese Doctor. The Usui system of Reiki is a very simple yet powerful form of healing which is easily given and received by anyone.

The word Reiki has its roots in two words: **Rei means universal and Ki means life force or energy.** Ki is the energy that all things are made of, like the Chinese Chi (as in Chi Gung or Tai Chi) and is the fundamental energy of everything physical and everything in other planes of consciousness.

Reiki is a special kind of healing energy that can only be channeled by someone who has been attuned to it. The attunement or initiation is the continuation of an ancient process of aligning the initiate with the Reiki healing energies using sacred Reiki symbols revealed to Dr. Usui. Once attuned the initiate is a channel for Reiki healing energy for life. Reiki energy is a healing energy that moves through the healer and is spiritually guided to the recipient. This never depletes the healer's own energy and in fact helps to energize and heal the healer. Since Reiki energy is spiritually guided it always goes to where it is needed; it can be considered as an intelligent energy.

All healing uses a universal energy to heal, however Reiki healing is guided for use only for the greater good. Reiki energy can never be abused or misused. People who practice healing prior to receiving a Reiki attunement will usually notice a change in energies. Once attuned, Reiki treatments are then given by the practitioner who simply needs the intent to heal and places his or her hands on the person to be healed. Whilst a number of easily learned hand positions are used on the recipient's body, the Reiki energy has a way of naturally flowing to where it is needed and therefore needs no conscious direction by the healer.

As a Healthcare Professional, you are using this natural healing method probably every day and literally with every patient you meet. This course will give you the tool to enhance this ability to the highest level. You can use it with your patients to enhance their health condition to the best possible healing status and even for yourself on every personal level to improve your self-development and reduce your daily stress and fatigue to the minimal level.

Chapter 4: History of Reiki

Reiki was one of such systems developed in Japan. The system was rooted in Tendai Buddhism and Shintoism.

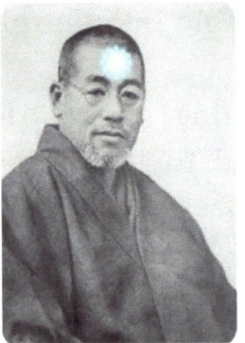

Dr. Usui

Founder and the first grand master.

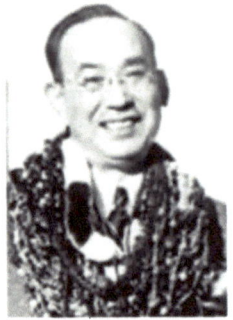

Dr. Hayashi

2nd grand master and organized reiki training and the all body treatments.

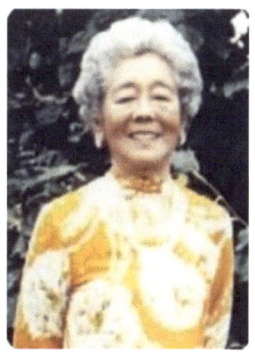

Madam Takata

3rd grand master, healed herself, studied and then took reiki to the west.

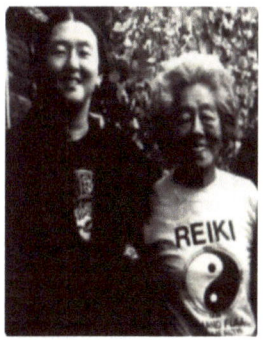

Furumoto

Granddaughter of madam Takata, formed Reiki Alliance.

Later Dr. Weber accredited for creating AIRA (the American International Reiki Association)

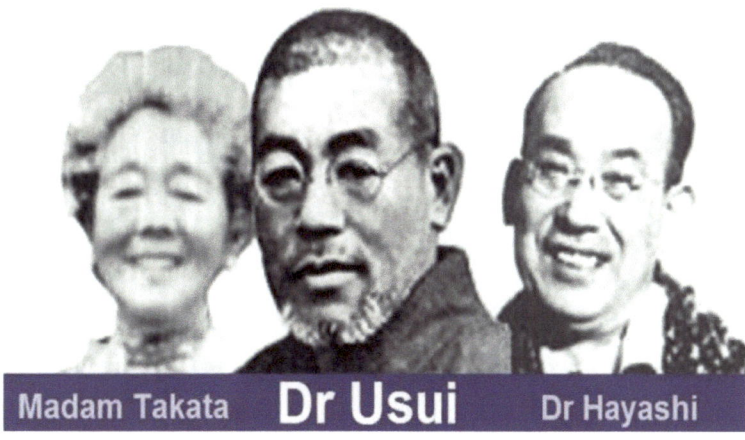

Madam Takata   Dr Usui   Dr Hayashi

Chapter 5: Legend of Dr. Mikao Usui

Dr. Mikao Usui was born in Japan 1865. He was a bright man of many talents who was looking for a spiritual path that would rekindle ancient traditions while embracing new ways. Reiki was one of such systems developed at this time in Japan.

The system was rooted in Tendai Buddhism and Shintoism. Usui was teaching his system long before he carried out the meditation.

He referred to his system as a "Method to Achieve Personal Perfection". According to Usui's Memorial stone, Usui was a well-known and popular healer. He would give his students empowerments to connect them to Reiki permanently. With this, they could treat themselves in between appointments with him. If they wanted to take things further they could begin an open-ended program of training in his system. Reiki was re-discovered by Dr. Mikao Usui, the founder of the Usui System of Reiki. Being an honorable Japanese man he decided to dedicate his life to discovering the inner healing powers and the ultimate purpose of life.

Dr. Usui was aware that there were many people around him unable to lead happy and productive lives because of illness and physical disability.

Dr. Usui had decided that he would go to the top of Mount Kori-yama, a sacred mountain, where he fasted and meditated, following the instructions in the formula, for 21 days.

To keep track of time on the mountain he set up 21 stones and each day he threw one stone away. On the 21st day, after tossing away all of the stones, he had still not received the healing power. It was still night and he stood up, thinking that he had failed in his quest. As he looked out toward the horizon he saw a point of light coming toward him.

Looking at the light he realized that it fact it has a consciousness and was communicating with him. He realized that the light contained the healing power that he was looking for but he also became aware that the light was so powerful that if it hit him it might kill him. He decided that the ability to heal was worth the risk and although he was afraid, he did not move.

The beam struck him on the forehead, knocking him unconscious. Rising out of his physical body he saw bubbles of light containing the sacred Reiki symbols. He immediately received an attunement and knowledge of each symbol and was, as a consequence, initiated into Reiki.

Dr. Usui hurried down the mountain. In his haste he fell over, stubbing his big toe and tearing the toe nail. He placed both of his hands over the injured area and within minutes the pain and the bleeding had stopped and shortly after he was completely healed. Having fasted for 21 days, he was very hungry, so when he reached the foot of the mountain he decided to stop at an inn for something to eat. While waiting for his meal to be cooked he heard a young girl crying in a house nearby.

Investigating, he found that the girl had been suffering for days with a bad toothache. Dr. Usui laid his hands on her face and within minutes the swelling receded and the pain stopped.

Dr. Usui continued to practice Reiki healing and before his death in 1926 had given the Reiki Master attunement to 16-18 people. Reiki was brought from Japan to the west during the second World War by Hawayo Takata and it is her Granddaughter, Phyllis Furumoto who is the current Reiki Grand Master. It is due to the incredible Divine aspirations of Dr. Usui and his compassionate desire to bring healing to people that this beautiful healing system has been rediscovered, formalized and spread around the world.

Eventually, Usui left the beggar's colony and started to teach people how to heal themselves. Usui practiced and taught Reiki throughout Japan for the remainder of his life, and passed on the Master attunement to 16 other disciples.
Before his death in the late 1920s he passed on the Master attunement to one of his students, Dr. Chujiro Hayashi.

Dr. Chujiro Hayashi

Chujiro Hayashi, born 1878, was a former Captain in the Imperial Navy, and a Naval Doctor. He took his Master training with Usui in 1925 at the age of 47.

He and two other Naval Officers, Ushida and Taketomi, were the last to be taught by Usui. Hayashi opened a clinic with eight beds and 16 healers, where clients would be treated by two or more healers. Hayashi kept a detailed record of the treatments, and used this information to create a manual of 'standard' hand positions for different ailments.

Hawayo Takata

Mrs. Hawayo Takata was born in 1900 on the island of Kauai, Hawaii. She suffered from serious medical conditions, and was about to undergo an operation. On the operating table, just before the surgery was about to start, Mrs. Takata heard a voice saying: "The operation is not necessary". She asked her doctor if he knew of any other ways to restore her health issue, and he referred her to Dr. Hayashi's clinic.

Mrs. Takata felt the heat from the practitioners' hands in Dr. Hayashi's clinic being so strong that she was sure they were using some sort of electrical equipment – maybe little electric heaters secreted up their sleeves. She looked into the large sleeves of their Japanese kimonos, and under the treatment table, but there was nothing there. Her skepticism turned to belief as her health problems resolved, and she decided that she wanted to learn Reiki.

At the same time Dr. Hayashi was looking to teach Reiki to another woman besides his wife, knowing that women would not be called up to fight in the war. Since Mrs. Takata was persistent he taught her to a Master level, in 1938, and gave her permission to teach Reiki in the West. She was the 13th and probably the last Reiki Master that Dr. Hayashi initiated. Between 1970 and her death in 1980 Mrs. Takata taught 22 Reiki Masters. Until quite recently, all Reiki practitioners in the West derived their Reiki from this lady.

Phyllis Lei Furumoto

Phyllis is Mrs. Takata's granddaughter, and received her First Degree initiation as a young child. However, it wasn't until she was 27 years old that she accepted the Second Degree initiation. Towards the end of the 1970s she was initiated as a Master, and worked with her grandmother on training others into Reiki. After Mrs. Takata's death the Western Reiki society split in two: 'The Reiki Alliance' led by Phyllis, and the 'Radiance Technique' led by Barbara Webber Ray. Barbara divided Reiki into seven degrees under the system she named 'The Radiance Technique'.

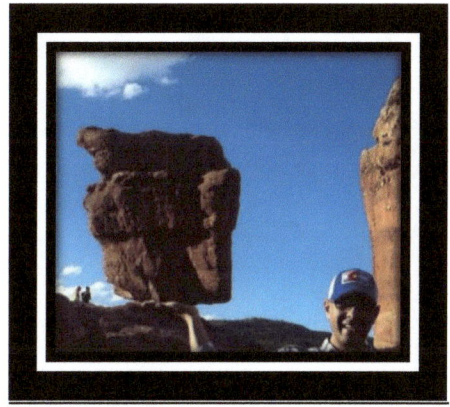

Chapter 6: The Reiki Principles

Learn the Gokai (Five Reiki Principles) in Japanese
The Gokai means the five principles in English. It was specially created by the founder of Reiki, Mikao Usui - to support our life, to be happier and healthier.

How does the Gokai work?

In Japan, traditionally they have a belief that the mystical powers dwell in words. This concept is called" Kototama". "Koto means "word" and "tama means "soul, spirit". The words we say has significant power. So day by day, we seed those words of Gokai into our life and it can influence our environment, body, mind, and soul. By chanting aloud, the energy of the words manifests in the world.

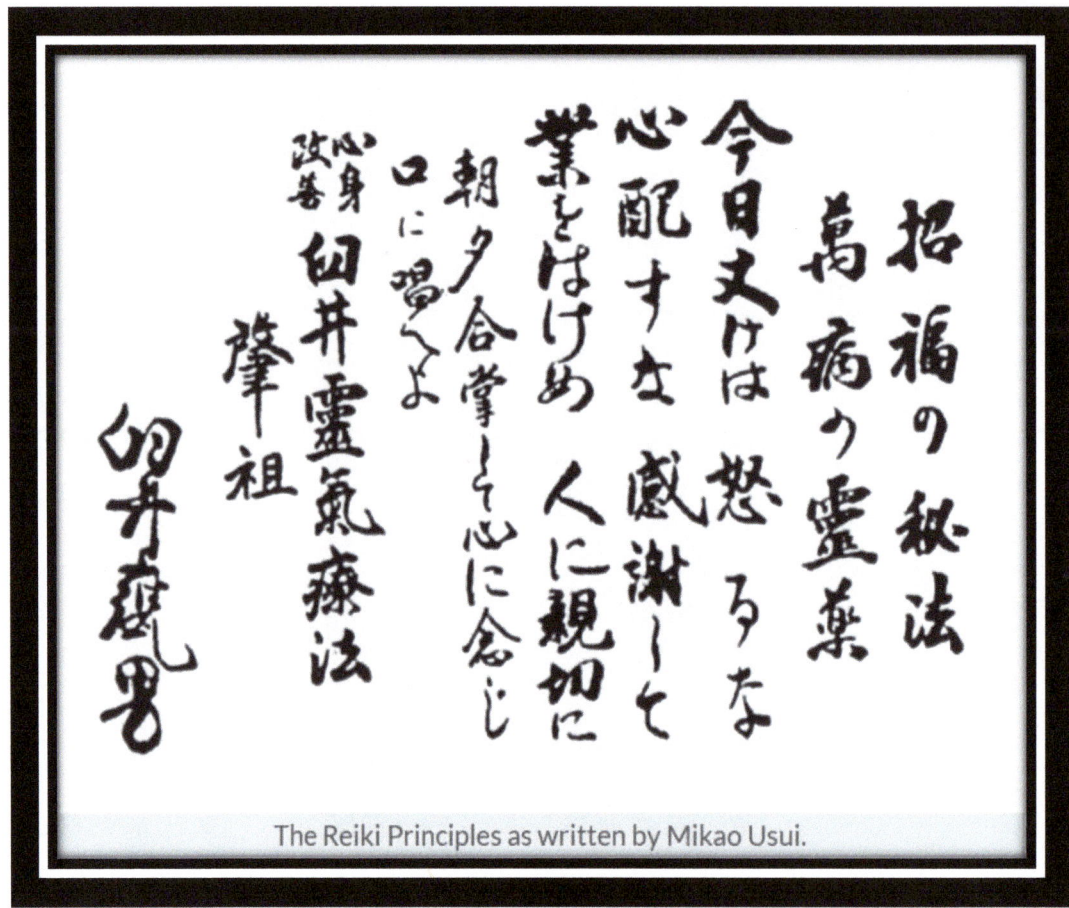

The Reiki Principles as written by Mikao Usui.

The 5 Reiki Principles

Just for Today (The 2 No's and 3 Be's)

<u>No</u> Worries (I will not worry)

<u>No</u> Anger (I will not be angry)

<u>Be</u> Honest (I will do my work honestly)

<u>Be</u> compassionate (I will give thanks for my many blessings)

<u>Be</u> Humble (I will be kind to every living thing)

Just for Today: I Will Not Worry!

Worries causes stress and anxiety; laughter is a wonderful; healer have fun life is too short to waste it worrying.

Hand Positions on the Heart and the Root Chakras to eliminate worries.

Just for Today: I Will Not Be Angry

Anger is a powerful emotion, when we get angry we lose control. We must understand triggers our anger. Take back control of your emotion. Choose to respond to situations in a positive way. Every time you meet or talk to someone there is an exchange of energy. Don't let them steel your energy. Anger is a choice response choose to live a healthier life free from Anger.

Hand Position on the 3rd Eye and the Root Chakras to eliminate Anger

Just for Today:

I Will Do My Work Honestly

Honesty means different things to different people, everyone at some point is dishonest, live every second in harmony and honesty with yourself and others.

Hand Position on the 3rd Eye and the Solar Chakras to enhance Honesty

Just for Today: I Will Give My Many Thanks for All My Blessings

Appreciate the many blessings in your life, count them if you can. That gives you the positive energy of diminish the negative feelings of you want to have something but you can't or it takes longer than you expect.

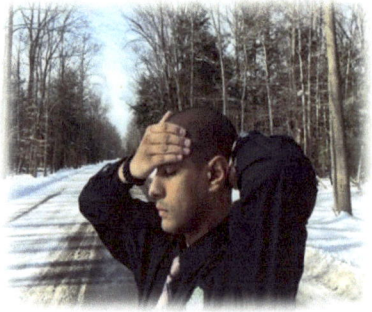

Hand Position on the 3rd Eye Chakra from the front and back to enhance Thankful

Just for Today: I Will Be Kind to My Neighbor and Every Living Thing

What goes around comes around. Karma is a two edge sword.

Hand Positions on first position the 3rd Eye & Throat Chakras, and Second position on the Heart & Root Chakras to enhance Humble and compassionate

It is important to remember that the Reiki principles are only guides for a happier and more fulfilling life. Use meditation to unlock the true meaning of these precepts and incorporate them into your life. They will help to transform your heart and soul.

They Are Not Commandments; They Are Gifts of Wisdom.

Section One Quiz- Introduction to Reiki

1. What are the three levels of Reiki?

2. The word Reiki is made up of two Japanese words, Rei and Ki. What does Rei mean?

3. Who was the founder of the Reiki system?

4. What does Ki mean?

5. How does Reiki promote healing?

6. What is Reiki?

7. True/False: Reiki creates deep relaxation and aids the body to release stress and tension?

8. What are the 5 Reiki Principles?

9. What is Gokai?

10. What is a chakra?

ANSWERS: #1. Level 1- Reiki Practitioner, Level II- Reiki Therapist, Level III – Reiki Master Teacher. #2. Universal life energy. #3. Dr. Usui #4. Life Force #5. Through relation and stress reduction #6. A Japanese healing technique. #7. True 8. See page 21 #9. The name of the 5 principles in Japanese. #10. Chakras are pathways for the energy to travel through our body.

Section 2: Energy Systems

Section 2

Chapter 8: Chakras

Reiki is the key that unlock the body's optimum capabilities, there are 7 main energy centers in the body called Chakras.

The 7 Major Chakra Points

*The Crown Chakra

*The Third Eye Chakra

*The Heart Chakra

*The Solar Plexus Chakra

*The Sacral Chakra

*The Root Chakra

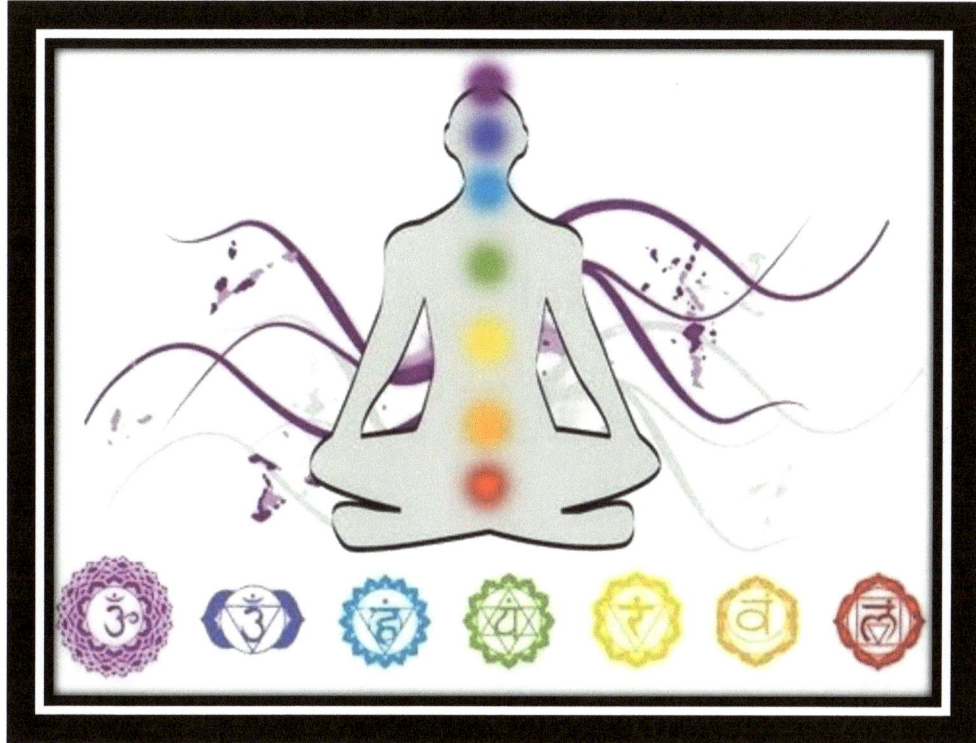

Chapter 9: Universal Life Force Energy Intuition

Reiki the Universal life force is nonphysical energy it is the Power to heal and influence our lives. Reiki Energy inside all of us, it is conception.

Reiki is conscious and consciousness is Love, therefore Reiki is Love Energy within every living thing. So, when you are using Reiki for healing with your patient you are sharing the universal life Love force energy to heal them, you are using your Intuition to guide you towards their body healing. It is extension to your daily practice with your patients either you are a Doctor, Nurse, health practitioner.

There is a different form of the universal life force energy like Reiki, Ta Chi, Feng Shui, Meditation, Yoga and Acupuncture. All of these are different forms of the universal life force energy and it is for your intuition to choose which one will help you to heal your patient the best.

10 things weaken the Life giving Energy:

1. Too much alcohol
2. A poor diet
3. A lack of exercises
4. Drugs
5. Tobacco
6. Negative habits
7. Stress
8. Poor breathing
9. Lack of sleeping and rest
10. Negative psychic activity

Humanity has become fragmented and hollow because of these 10 bad habits and more, your natural abilities to heal yourself and others are here and now. Help your patients to feel better by this natural ability you have and everybody has. Teach them how they can heel themselves too.

More wisdom and growth in your self-development means happier and fulfilling life.

Everyone has access to Reiki we all use Reiki daily.

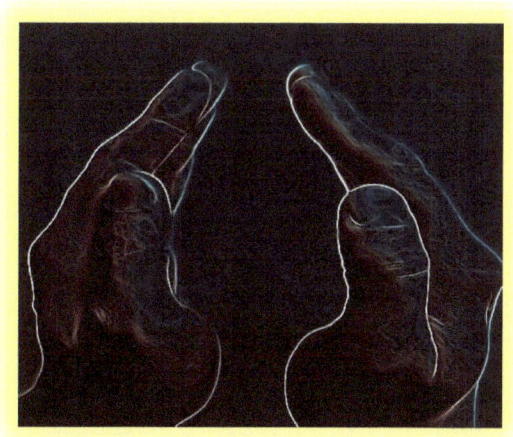

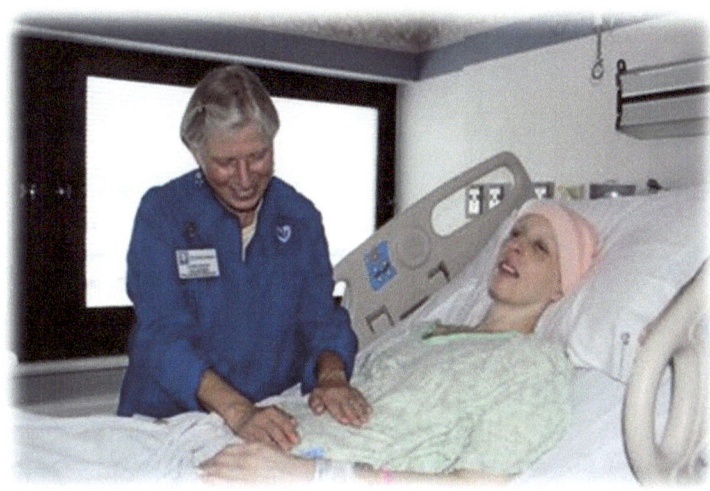

This Wonderful Reiki Energy is FREE and Abundant

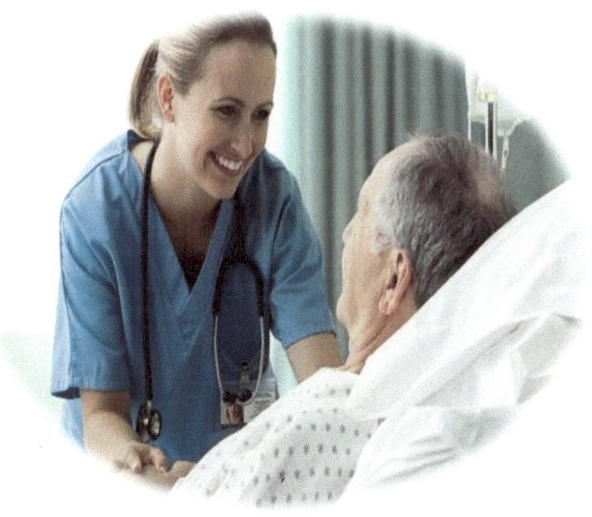

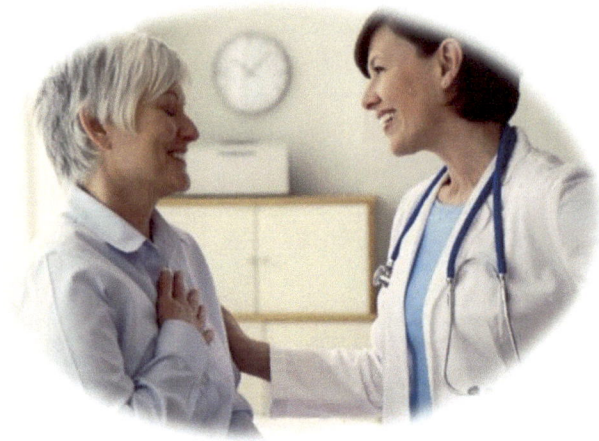

Reiki is part of our genetic structure, Reiki stimulates growth, health, life and healing.

"Reiki is the greatest secret in the science of energetics."

Madam Hawayo Takata

Chapter 10: Wave form of Life

(Ultradian Rhythm Technique)

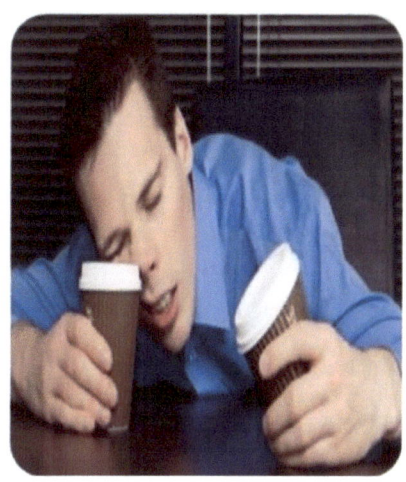

Waveform of Life

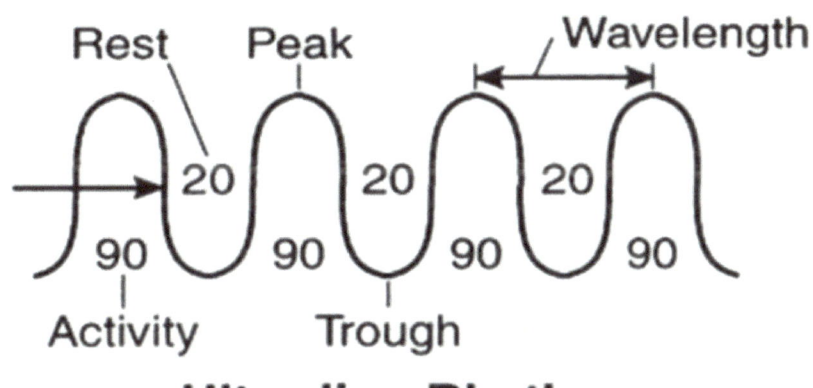

Ultradian Rhythm

Ultradian rhythms and the natural 'trance cycle'

You may have heard of the 'Circadian rhythm' the daily bodily cycle that regulates our 'awakeness' during the day and night. The Circadian rhythm is the reason that we feel like getting up in the morning (hopefully!) and what causes us to feel sleepy at bedtime. Another type of bodily rhythm is the

'Ultradian' rhythm. Whereas the circadian rhythm occurs once a day, ultradian rhythms happen more than once.

One ultradian rhythm has been shown to moderate the 'hemispheric dominance' within the brain. Although the exact function and interplay of the 2 hemispheres is as yet unknown, we do know that the left hemisphere is more specialized for linear, logical thought and communication, and the right is more active when we are relaxed, dreaming and in hypnosis. If not too stressed, you will have, after getting out of bed in the morning, around 90 to 120 minutes more focused attention followed by a 20-minute period of lesser focus. This is often experienced as difficulty concentrating. During this 20-minute period you are more likely to feel sleepy or 'day dreamy' This is often the time that people take a break, grab a coffee or smoke a cigarette as away to try and cheat this natural break. However, since it has been shown that taking advantage of this natural rhythm has profound physical and mental health benefits, it is a better idea to do what your brain is asking you to do, Relax! Being able to use Reiki at these times is a highly efficient way of relaxing quickly and deeply and maximizing the benefit to your body and mind.

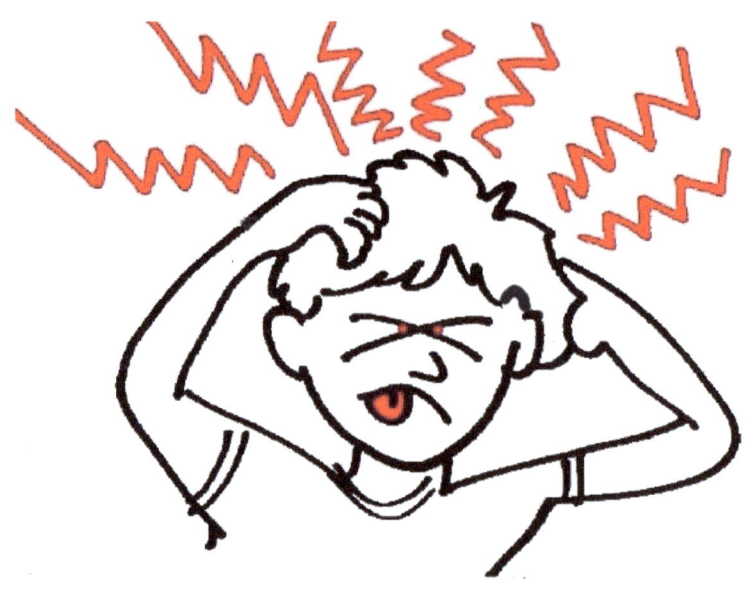

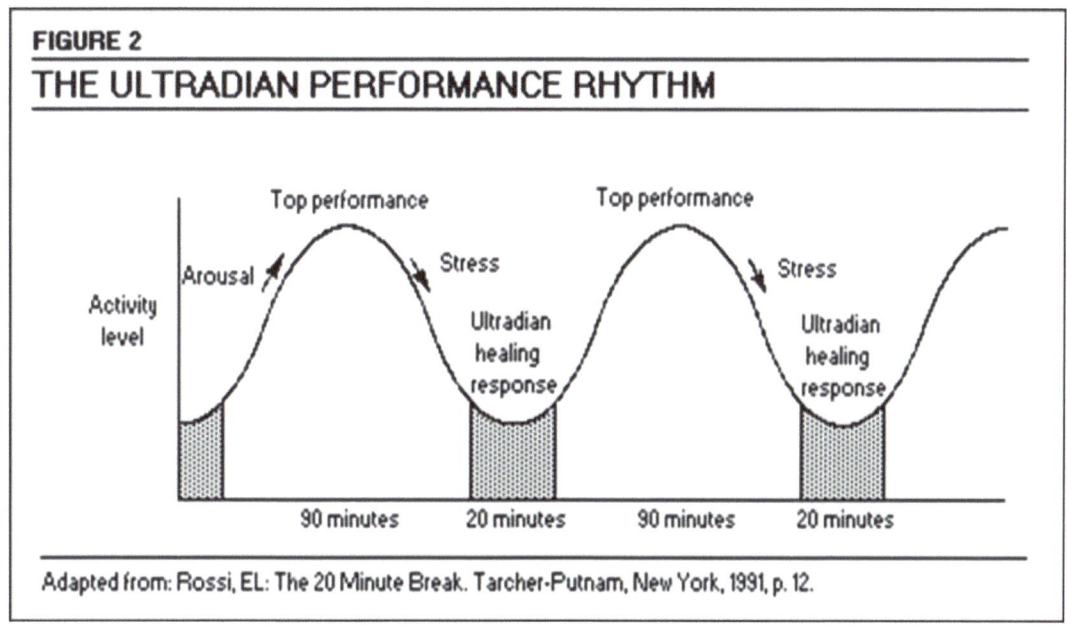

FIGURE 2

THE ULTRADIAN PERFORMANCE RHYTHM

Adapted from: Rossi, EL: The 20 Minute Break. Tarcher-Putnam, New York, 1991, p. 12.

Neglect can lead to health problems.

Reiki can be used to rebalance the body mind and spirit.

<u>Solution?</u>

Look out for signs that you need a short break.

Cup hands over eyes and go inside send healing Reiki!

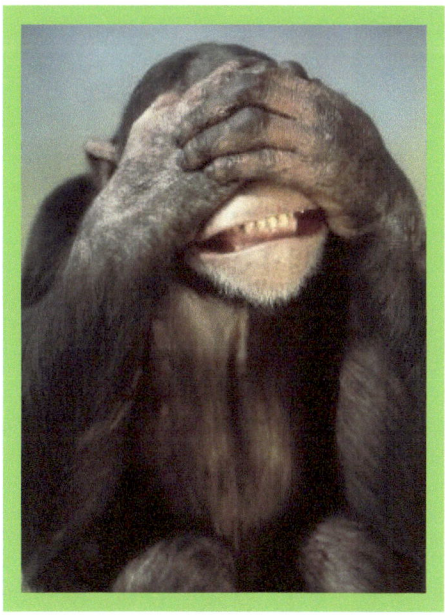

If time is an issue you can use another quick energy boosting technique

The thymus gland works with your immune system.

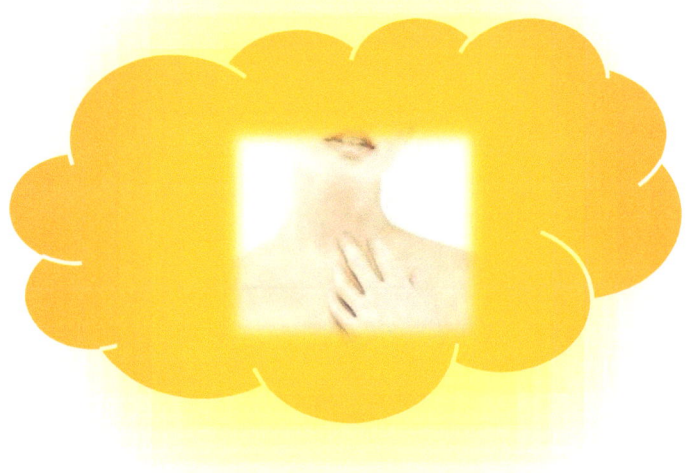

- **Tap gently 20-30 times on the area of the area of the thymus gland You can also place your hand over the area to boost your energy and immune system. (Pretty Cool!)**

"Your body's ability to heal is greater than anyone has permitted you to believe!"

-Unknown

"Natural Forces Within Us are the True Healers of Disease."

-Hippocrates

Section Two Quiz: Energy Systems

1. What are the 7 major chakra points?
2. Name something that can weaken the life giving energy?
3. What is Ultradian rhythms and when is a good time to use Reiki with Ultradian rhythms?
4. What technique can you do to boost your energy level?
5. True/False- Reiki will work on all living things?

ANSWERS: #1. The Crown, Third Eye, Heart, Solar Plexus, Sacral and Root Chakra's. #2. Alcohol, exercise, diet, drugs, tobacco, stress etc. #3. Ultradian is body rhythm it moderates the 'hemispheric dominance' within the brain. When you feel sleepy or day dreaming is the best time to use Reiki. #4. The best technique is to tap on the thymus gland to boost energy. #5. True- Reiki works on all living things including pets and

Section 3: Performing a Reiki Session

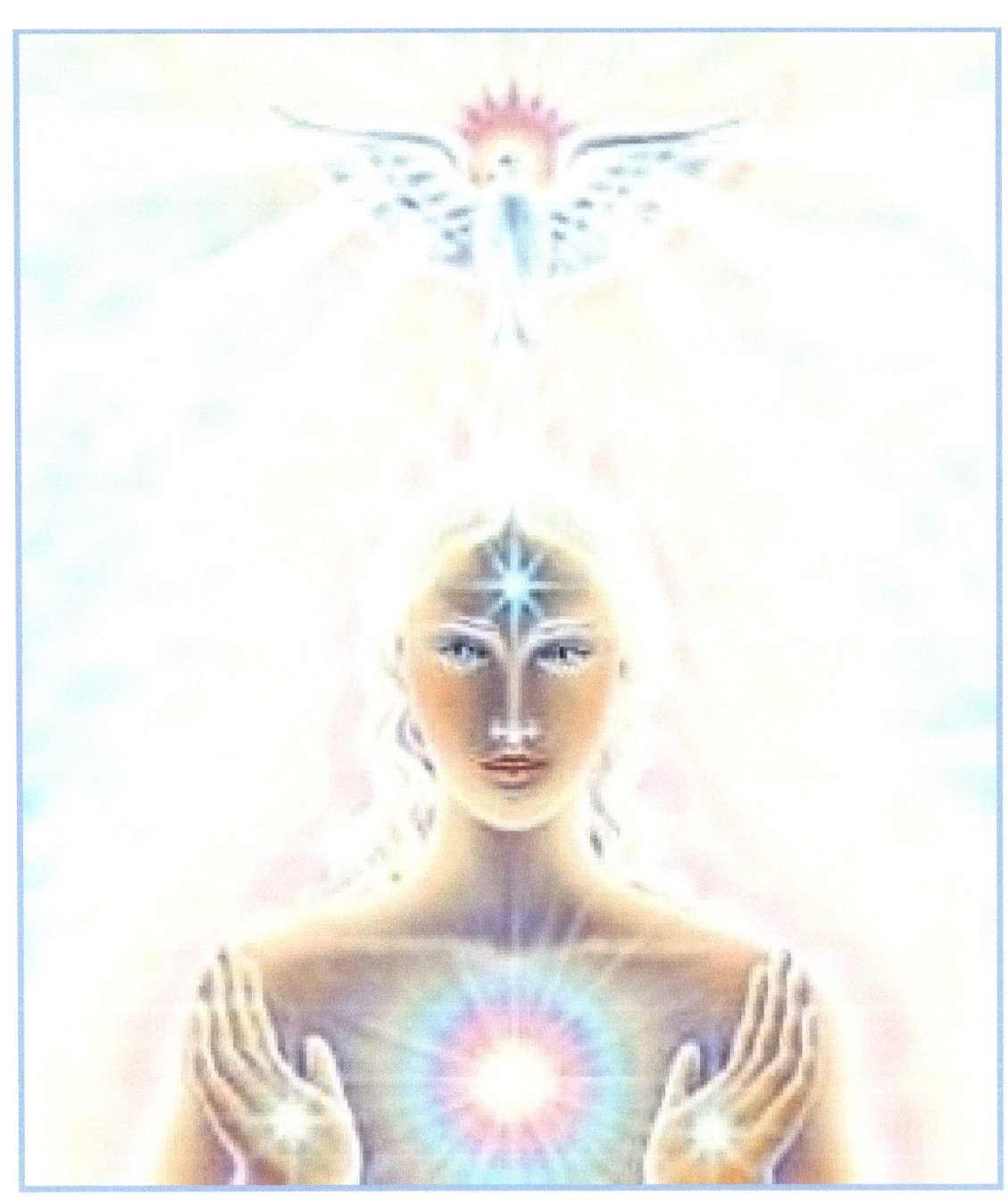

Chapter 12: Preparing to Use Reiki

Reiki is simple and easy to learn; the results is profound. Reiki will bring the recipients mind body and spirit into balance.

Madam Takata described Reiki as being similar to radio waves, cannot see the waves that are everywhere.

Reiki Attunement

(Initiation Ceremony)

Reiki attunement means to be Tuned into Reiki.

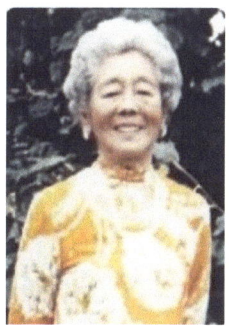

Reiki is ever present in your body, the Attunement adds balance and increases energy level and capacity.

Reiki stays with us for life, reiki is pure energy, reiki is channeled through the hands.

Ways to use Reiki after attunment

Use reiki on every thing!

You are only limited by your imagination!

"Reiki is Love,

Love is Wholeness,

Wholeness is Balance,

Balance is Well Being

Well Being is Freedom from Disease." – Dr. Mikao Usui

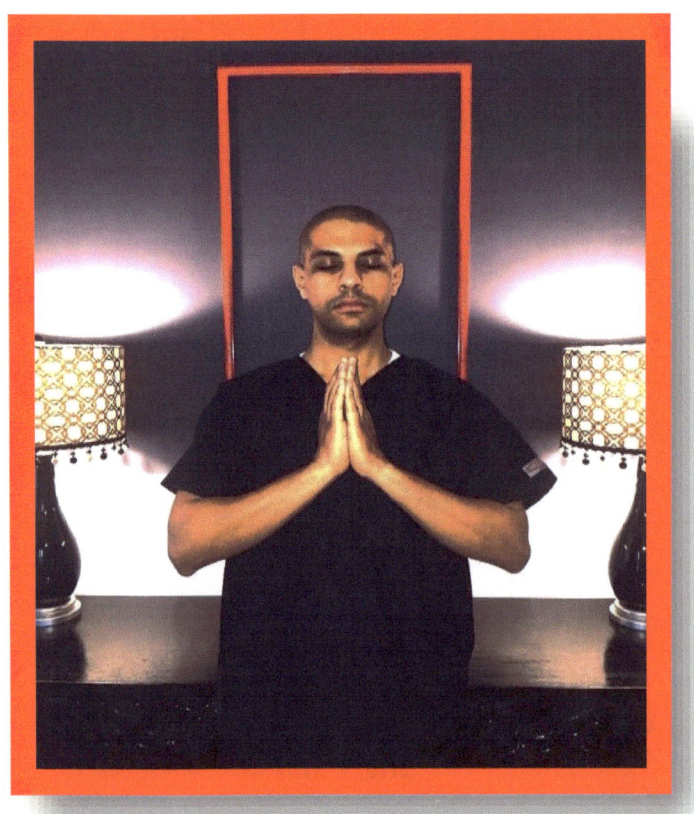

Reiki Level I - Attunements

The Reiki first degree attunements connect you to the Reiki source and allow healing energy to flow through you. The attunements are passed by a Reiki Master in a sacred ceremony that connects upper chakras and the chakras in the palms of the hands to the Reiki source using sacred Reiki symbols. This attunement does not take very long; it does not hurt and it lasts for life. The attunement process is divinely guided so that it is always done perfectly.

The Effects of the Reiki I Attunements

The attunement has different effects on people but generally speaking people feel the effects of being healed and having their energies raised. A very few people may experience some flu-like symptoms afterwards, but this is really nothing to worry about. Some people may have spiritual experiences – feelings or visions or may feel elated at various times. For about the first three weeks after the attunements (The body Cleansing –is like a detoxification period) the initiate is being healed and cleared as a channel for the healing energy and so Reiki healers may feel some effects during this period.

Things to Do After You Have Been Attuned: Reiki Level I

I recommend that for the three weeks following the attunements initiates should meditate every day, even if for only a short while. Meditating on the Reiki energies and asking for help in understanding and gaining insight into Reiki healing will be useful. The attunements have different effects on different people and initiates should follow their intuition as to what to do; you may feel that you need do nothing. Saying prayers - asking for blessings from the Reiki Masters, Teachers and Guides is something that I would recommend.

I strongly recommend that Reiki I initiates give themselves a daily healing. I found this difficult at first and some will feel the energies flowing more than others, but this really is the best way to improve the power of your healing and to heal yourself. Persevere with giving yourself a daily Reiki treatment, even if it is not a full treatment, since this will initiate and sustain change and healing at all levels of your being.

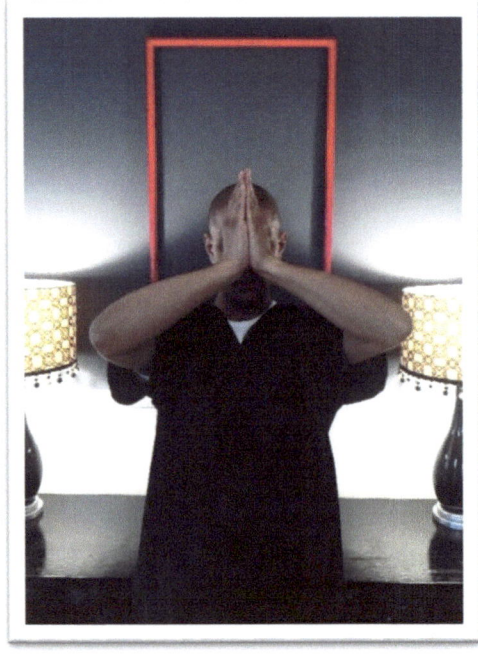

Notes:

Chapter 13: Student Testimonials About Their Attunement Experience

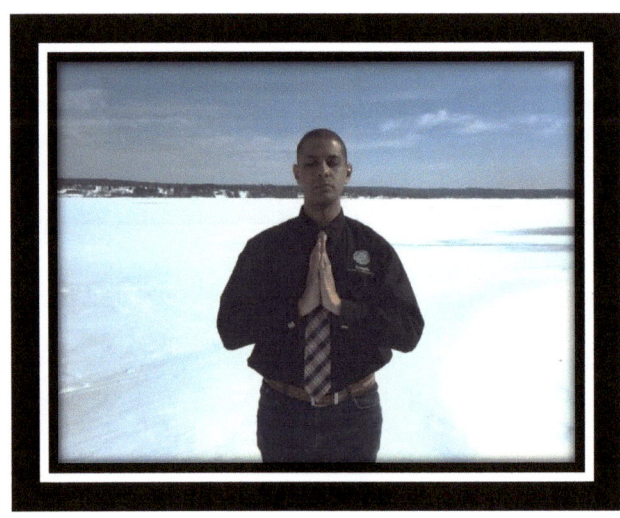

Notes:

(Please write your own experience before, during, & after the attunement)

Chapter 14: Anatomy for Reiki

(This section provides you with basic information regarding anatomy and physiology)

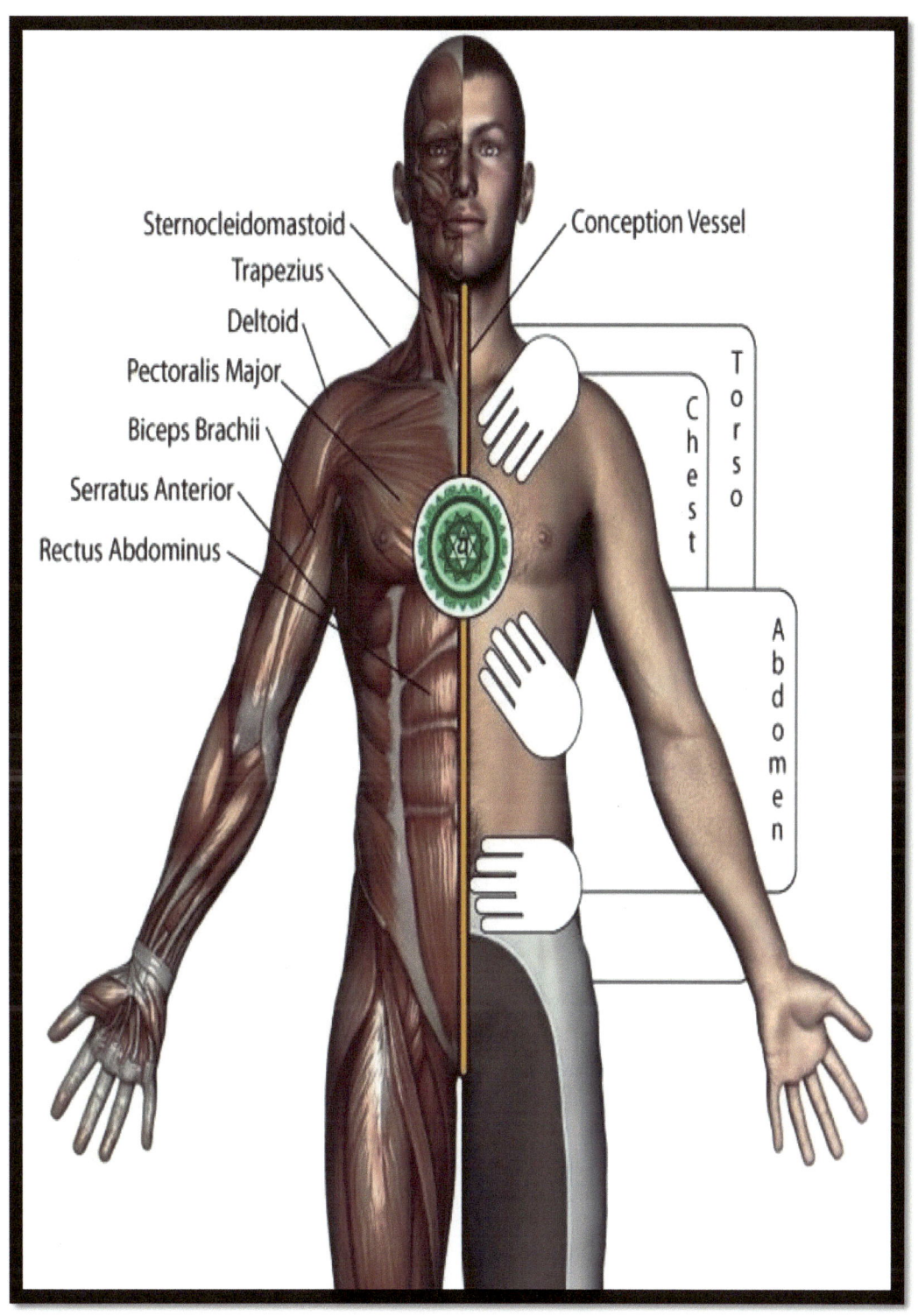

Lymphatic   Respiratory   Digestive   Urinary   Reproductive
System   System   System   System   System

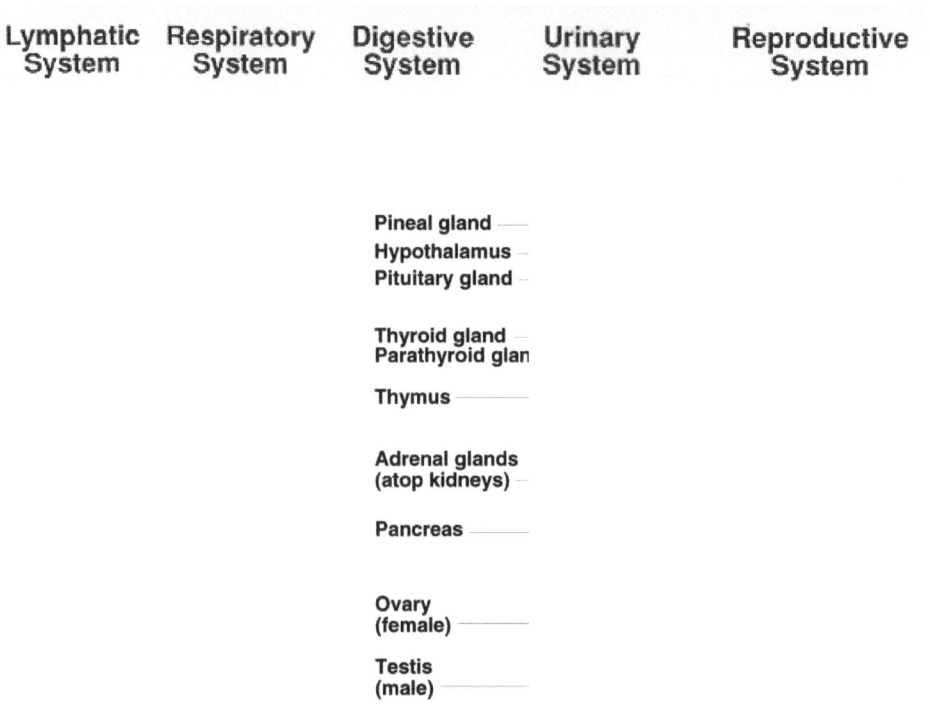

Pineal gland
Hypothalamus
Pituitary gland

Thyroid gland
Parathyroid glan

Thymus

Adrenal glands
(atop kidneys)

Pancreas

Ovary
(female)

Testis
(male)

Endocrine system

Ductless glands that release hormones.

Works tighter with the nervous system and regulates metabolic activities maintaining homeostasis.

Lymphatic system

System of thin tubes that runs thought-out the body.

Lymph plays an important role in the immune system and in absorbing fats from the intestines.

What is ATP?

ATP $=$ Adenosine + Energy + P$_i$ + Energy + P$_i$ + Energy + P$_i$

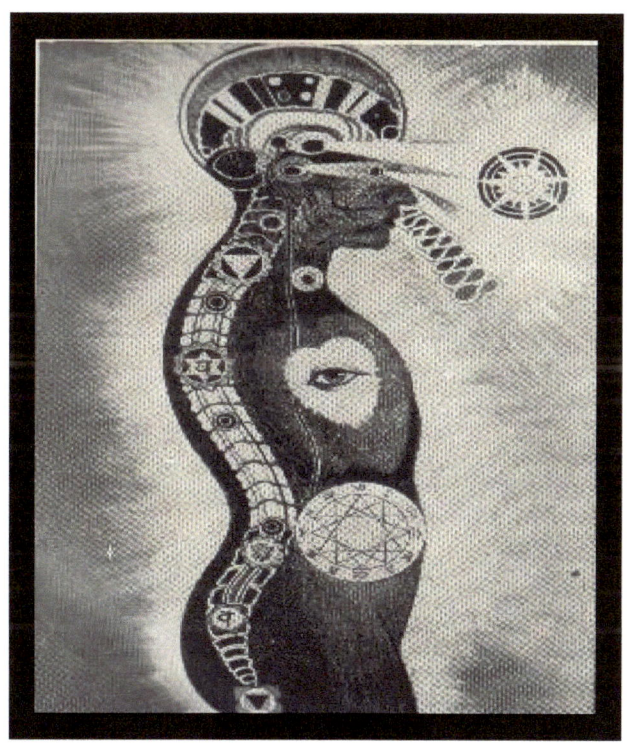

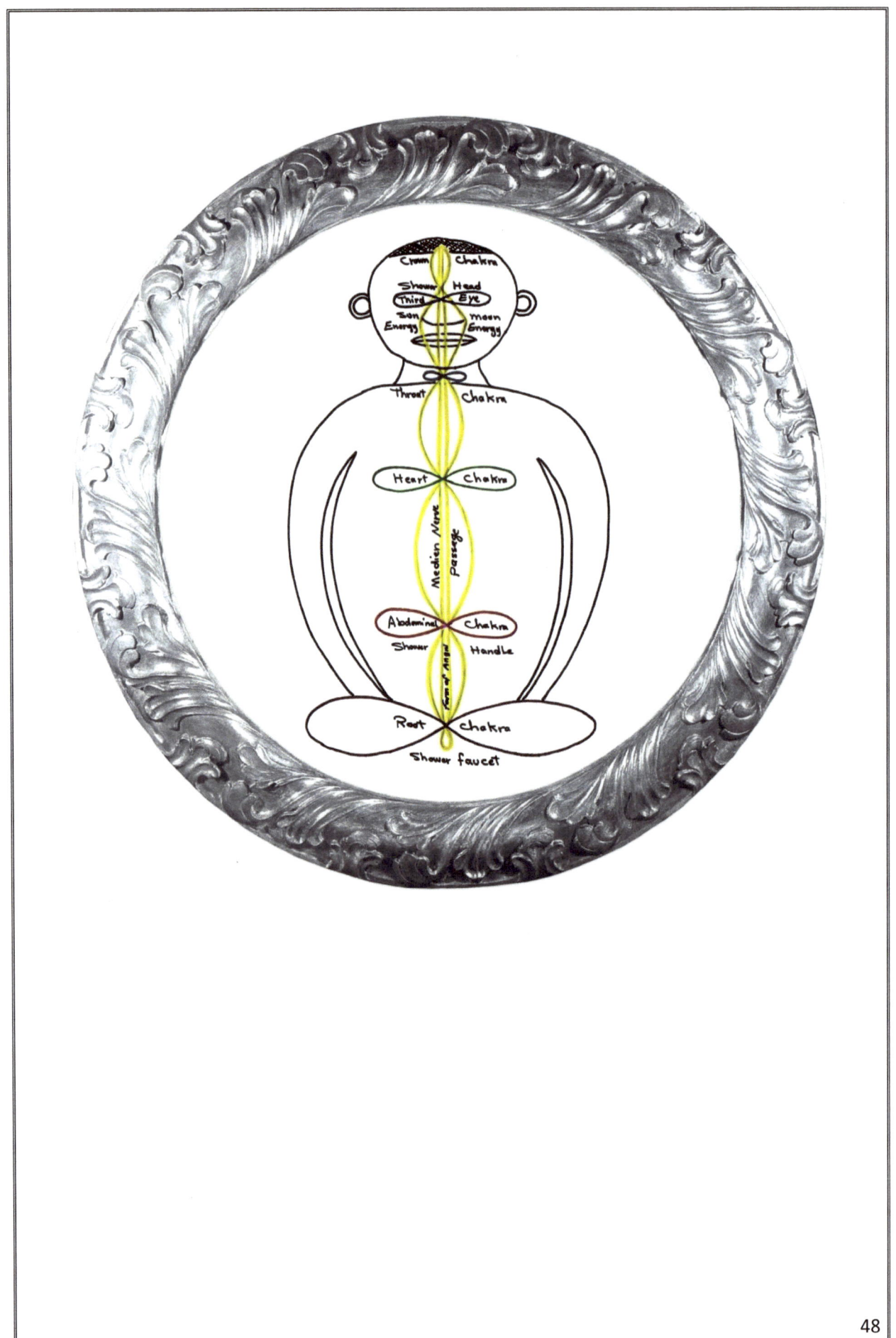

Chapter 15: Reiki Self-Treatments

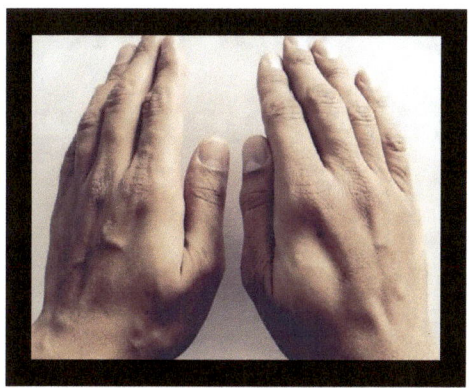

Reiki Treatment

Reiki treatment can feel like a wonderful glowing radiance that flows through you and surrounds you. As the hands are placed systematically on the body, and the 22 positions are held for anything from 3-10 minutes in any one place, the recipient can feel heat, ranging from hot to warm to cool. Some people feel gentle tingling in the hands or feet, while others feel strong waves of energy surging through the body. The stomach often rumbles as the energy flows through the system.

Sometimes a release of emotions can occur and tears will flow, irritation might appear or there may be a laugh of relief, or the recipient may fall asleep.

Reiki will work in whatever way the recipient needs it most, and this explains why students report differing experiences during the attunement process. Some students experience visions, or receive messages, healing, or past-life images during this very special time.

The majority of people find that it is an extremely relaxing experience.

"I saw colors"
"I felt very nurtured and loved"
"Your hands felt so warm"
"I could feel tingling in my fingers and toes"
"I feel that I am not afraid anymore to face my problems" "I felt very heavy on the couch"
"I now understand what I need to do next in my life" "I felt disorientated"
"Old memories came"

To practice Reiki, you need no special faith or belief system. While Reiki is spiritual in nature, it is not a religion. It has no dogma, and there is nothing you must believe in to learn and use it. Reiki is used by many faiths and religions as well as free thinkers and followers of many differing philosophies. While it has nothing to do with any religion it can enhance a person's religious beliefs by giving them a greater feeling of connectedness to the source.

Response

A 'healing response' can occur in days or weeks following healing. It is traditional within Reiki to think in terms of a 21-day period of clearing out or cleansing, as the energy starts to work on you.

Each person is different and so Reiki can have different effects. A healing response is healthy sign that the toxins in the body are being released. With the release of toxics there may be slight side effects, which usually last for about three days. It is quite important to drink plenty of water.

Sometimes there is an acceleration of the condition following a treatment, and this is a positive sign that the energy is working through the system.

During a treatment or shortly afterwards, it is possible that 'old' conditions may re-emerge. This is because the moving energy is breaking down toxins, which will normally disappear quite quickly.

It is important to remember that Reiki **can never harm**. Each person draws exactly what he or she needs at that time. Remember that we cannot direct Reiki to specific conditions and that it may work in a way that is unexpected. The client may not be relieved of the condition, something that they expected or hoped for, but may find that other benefits may have occurred, such as an emotional release or improvement in a condition that they have had for a long time and have become used to. Whatever healing occurs will be for the person's highest good. People often ask how many treatments they should have. Ideally, three treatments close together, on consecutive days.

Healing using Reiki

Reiki healing is always for the greatest good; it can never be abused or misused. Reiki healing goes to where it is needed, so it does not need to be directed. Reiki healing can work on every part of a person, of their body, mind and soul; it works on every chakra and every emotion; it works on their spirit and their karma. It can go to their past, present or future. Reiki healing can go to every part of a person, to every relationship of theirs and to every part of their life. Just trust that it is going to exactly where it is needed.

Reiki healing is always for the greatest good, even if we do not know what that is. If the Reiki healing that you give to yourself or someone else is not needed at that time, it is never wasted since it will be sent at a later time.

Self-healing

Through your intent to find out about yourself and to be healed and happy and through your commitment to change you have started the journey of self-healing. Through faith and trust in your divine guidance a load is lifted from your shoulders and you will know that you are going in the right direction.

The healing process itself can contain moments of exquisite love and joy and may even have times of deep pain and sadness. Changes will happen in your life: many small ones and some larger and more daunting but all changes will take you to a place of more happiness than you have known in your life.

Engaging the truth and finding out that we actually have nothing to fear is like taking off a huge suit of armor. It is removing the protection that we put in place due to our fear, the barriers that have kept out a great deal of life but have not actually made us more secure because our fear is on the inside. Once the armor is taken off we can breathe more easily, see more clearly, feel the pleasure of the sun and the wind and be liberated from our self - imposed imprisonment.

Many people suffer considerable trauma in their lives at some time and old wounds are another part of us that can be healed. The pain of separation from loved ones through bereavement or for other reasons can have a profound effect on people, as can any traumatic event. We all have coping mechanisms for such trauma that can often entail closing off a part of ourselves deep inside and this can be a subconscious self -protection measure. This protection can stay in place and the pain can stay buried until we undertake self-healing. The protection measure can keep a certain part of us blocked up and closed off and this is often exhibited as insecurity, an unwillingness to give or receive love or an inability to indulge in certain feelings, emotions or relationships.

Once you have been attuned to Reiki it is easy to give yourself Reiki healing; all that you do is use the hand positions to give yourself a treatment every day, if possible. This, together with your commitment to change and progression will heal you.

Chapter 16: Preparing to Work with Others & Healing Someone Else

It is not necessary to know about a person's attitudes and beliefs in order to give them healing and they do not have to be prepared to change them in order to receive healing however it obviously makes a huge difference. Know that just by showing someone love and compassion you are helping them and effectively giving them healing and if someone wants to receive healing you are helping them just by the act of giving unconditionally. At the level of Reiki 1 you can give healing to friends and family and know that by this act of kindness and attention you are helping them and helping your relationships with them.

But be prepared to go into a slightly different mode when you start healing with them. Try to put to one side the emotions that may naturally occur in your relationship. Create an appropriate atmosphere and a sacred space and wash your hands before and after healing.

Explain to your recipient what you will do and put them at their ease. Tell them that the Reiki energy is an intelligent energy and that they will get just the right amount of healing. Get their permission to lay your hands on them and make sure that you do not intrude upon their body or space. Whether the recipient is lying down or sitting in a chair, there is no problem if they drift off to sleep.

Giving Treatments to Others

Once you have been attuned to Reiki, you only need to place your hands on someone and the energy will flow automatically to the areas of need. It knows where to go. If you try to 'force' the process by 'willing' the recipient to get better, your ego starts to get in the way and there might be lessening in the power. You can 'draw down energy from above', though, in a neutral and way, to help increase the flow. Remember that you are a channel for the energy and that you are not the source of the healing. This explains why treatments do not drain you at all, but actively replenish and invigorate you. It is not your energy that you are dealing with. Before treating others wash your hands, and wash once again after giving the treatment. Suggest your client to take off their shoes and glasses, and loosen any restricting clothes if needed. Make sure your client is warm and comfortable on the treatment bed. Place your hands on your client slowly and gently. When removing your hands do so in slow movements.

When your hands are over your client's face, be careful not to press on their eyelids or against their nostrils. When working on the client's neck, take care not to let the weight of your hands rest on their throat. Do not lean on your client or apply undue pressure. Do not try to force the outcome; just let the energy flow.

Placing Your Hands

With your Reiki 1 attunement you need, as much as possible to actually place your hand on the person: however, this will always need to be done with respect to the recipient's body and their personal space. Ask your client before you start healing or during the session whether they feel comfortable with your hands in certain positions. You should be aware what is acceptable and ask your client to be explicit about what they feel comfortable with and what they don't. Apply discretion. Where it may be suitable to place a hand on the front of a man's chest it would not be suitable with a woman. Equally the base chakra is a place which often needs a lot of work but where no hands can be placed. The way to overcome any awkwardness or embarrassment is to clearly ask the healing recipient and agree with them, before the session which areas may be touched and which may not.

There are set hand positions that Dr. Usui detailed for Reiki healing and these tend to be over the chakras, with additions. There are more hand positions around the head since this is an area of major importance. These are basic hand positions but you should be guided as to where to place your hands. You should also be guided as to how long to keep your hands in one position, but remember that Reiki healing flows to where it is most needed, so it is better to spend longer in the positions that are most comfortable and have the most contact with both hands. If you are healing for around three-quarters of an hour, then it may be suitable to spend at least ten minutes on the head. Use your intuition and divine guidance to sense where you should place your hands. If your client complains of a bad knee you may feel that you should spend time with your hands on their knee but you may also feel guided to return to the heart chakra and give more healing, there.

Intuitive working

Once you had some practice with treating other people, Reiki will increase its guidance in your treatment sessions – guiding you to specific areas in the client's body. This will happen as long as you are open to the possibility of working intuitively. This is not essential though. Don't worry if you end up doing most treatments following the 'standard' hand positions, because it will still work.

Approach your treatments with a neutral state of mind and do not try to 'force it' or impose your preferred solution on the situation. Simply let the energy flow and trust that it is going to the right place.

Scanning

To practice scanning, let your hand or hands hover over the person's body. Perhaps it would be better to start using one hand only. Move your hand(s) slowly over the body – you can be quite brisk, but not too quick so as not to miss the sensations. Focus your attention on the sensations you are experiencing in your palm and fingers and notice any changes or intensification of the sensation. As you scan, Reiki will guide you to the areas where it is most needed.

Ending the Treatment

Smooth down the aura - Make a number of sweeps over the recipient's body, moving from the crown to the feet (not the other direction). Intend to smooth the energy field all-round the client's body, front and back.

Disconnect -

At the beginning of a treatment you have tuned yourself to the recipient, so at the end of treatment you should disconnect. Many practitioners will shake their hands or rub their hands together, or blow through them, or a combination of the above.

The 'Dantien'

The Dantien is an energy center located two fingerbreadths (3-5 cm) below your tummy button and 1/3 of the way into your body. It is your personal energy store, the focus of your personal power, which is used in a variety of oriental techniques. It is also seen as the center of your intuition and your creativity, so when people carry out Japanese calligraphy, or Ikebana (flower arranging) and the Tea ceremony, they are focusing their attention on the Dantien. The Dantien, a Chinese word, is referred to as the **'Tanden'** in Japanese.

Reiki First Degree Techniques

The following techniques are taught in Reiki One course:

Hatsu Rei Ho (warming up!)

Hatsu Rei Ho is designed to be carried out every day for 10-15 minutes.
The Japanese word 'Hatsu Rei' means 'start up Reiki' 'Ho' means 'technique'.

Kenyoku (Dry Bathing)

Kenyoku can be carried out at the beginning and end of a treatment as a way of disconnecting you from unwanted energies in your surroundings, from your patient, and from your thoughts. It can be used to protect yourself from worrisome or stressful situations, to stop things from bothering you, and to stop you from 'bringing work home'.

Gassho

Gassho means 'hands together', and the correct position is to have your hands together in front of your chest (like praying hands), just above your heart, so that you can breathe out onto your fingertips. Hold this position for meditation.

Focus your awareness on the point where your middle fingers touch. You can try touching with your tongue the roof of your mouth with each in-breath, and let the tongue go down, with each out-breath. See if that makes any difference for you.

Energy exercises

Here are some exercises that you can carry out to experience the energy and build up your sensitivity. You will need a partner for some of them.

Feel Energy between your hands

Rub your hands together for half a minute. Hold your hands out in front of you, shoulder width apart, with your palms facing each other.

Now slowly 'bounce' your hands together until you feel an impression of something tangible between your hands. You may feel something squashy like a marshmallow, a balloon or a rubber ball; you may feel a surface, a layer, some resistance, some magnetic repulsion... some 'thing' that your hands are resting on, and which prevents them from touching each other. You are feeling your energy field, which was always there for you. To be aware of it and experience it you have simply focused your attention...

Feel a Rainbow between your hands

Rub your hands together for half a minute. Hold your hands, your palms facing up. Try to feel a Rainbow of color, with its right 'leg' on your right palm, and its left 'leg' on your left palm. Try to move your hand to see if the

Rainbow expands.

Now, try to 'hand over' your partner one leg of the Rainbow, keeping the other leg on your palm. The Rainbow now goes from you to your partner. What colors do you see? Is there any movement of energy? Does it move from you to your partner, or from them back to you?

Feel Energy on a partner's hand

Sit fairly near your partner. Rub your hands for half a minute. Hold one hand out in front of you, at shoulder height, with your palm facing your partner's palm, rather like you were about to push his/her hand away from you.

Now slowly 'bounce' your hands together until you have an impression that there is something tangible between your hands.

See if you can agree between yourselves about the point where you can both feel that 'contact', an energy presence or surface that may feel like magnetic resistance.
Now one person should keep their hand still while the other person slowly moves their hand vertically up and down, from side to side, and slowly towards and away from their partner's palm. How does this feel? What sensations are you experiencing? How do the sensations change?

Feel Energy on a partner's head & shoulders

One person sits and closes their eyes. You stand behind them and raise your hands, palms down, hovering about 30 cm above the other person's head. Now bring your hands slowly down, bouncing them down until you feel that your hands are resting on your partner's energy field. Move your hands away again and 'bounce' them down onto an adjacent area above the head. Feel the energy field over different parts of the partner's head, the forehead, the back of the head and the temples.

Push someone off balance using Energy

Your partner should stand up, standing still with their eyes closed. They should not stand stiff, but relaxed. If they feel that their body wants to drift either forwards or backwards then they should not resist, but simply allow their body to drift naturally. If they need to take a step back to steady themselves then they can do so.

Stand about two meters behind the person with your hands in front of your chest, palms facing away from you and towards your partner, as if you were going to push their shoulders. Slowly move towards them until you have an impression that your hands are resting on the person's energy field.

You may have some physical sensations or you may simply 'know' that your hands have made contact with the person's energy field.

Now, try to 'pull' their energy field away from their body for 20-30 seconds, by moving your palms away from their body. You can take a step back, or even a few steps back, and you can imagine that their energy field is being stretched out like an elastic field, being pulled away.

Do not alternate quickly between pushing and pulling. You need to be either squashing their energy field for a while, or pulling it away for a while. Your body is used to being in the center of its energy field, and if you distort that field then your body seems to want to drift into a position to balance.

Play with Energy Balls

Hold your hands approximately 22 cm apart and imagine that energy is flooding through your palms into the space between. You are building up a ball of energy between your hands. Bounce your hands against this ball of energy and feel it becoming stronger and denser over a period of a couple of minutes. When you feel ready, slowly pass the energy ball to someone sitting next to you and place it gently in their hands.

Self-healing is the starting point.

Reiki is always available to you.

Possibilities are endless the benefits immeasurable.

Reiki can help you!

Reiki works holistically on the mind, body & spirit.

How to treat yourself with reiki?

No right no wrong.

Hand positions are only a guide use your intuition!

The areas of the body to treat specific ailments described by the founder of Reiki, Mikao Usui (1865-1926), were loosely inspired by the prevalent scientific medicine in that culture and era: Traditional Chinese Medicine.

Self Healing

Hand Positions

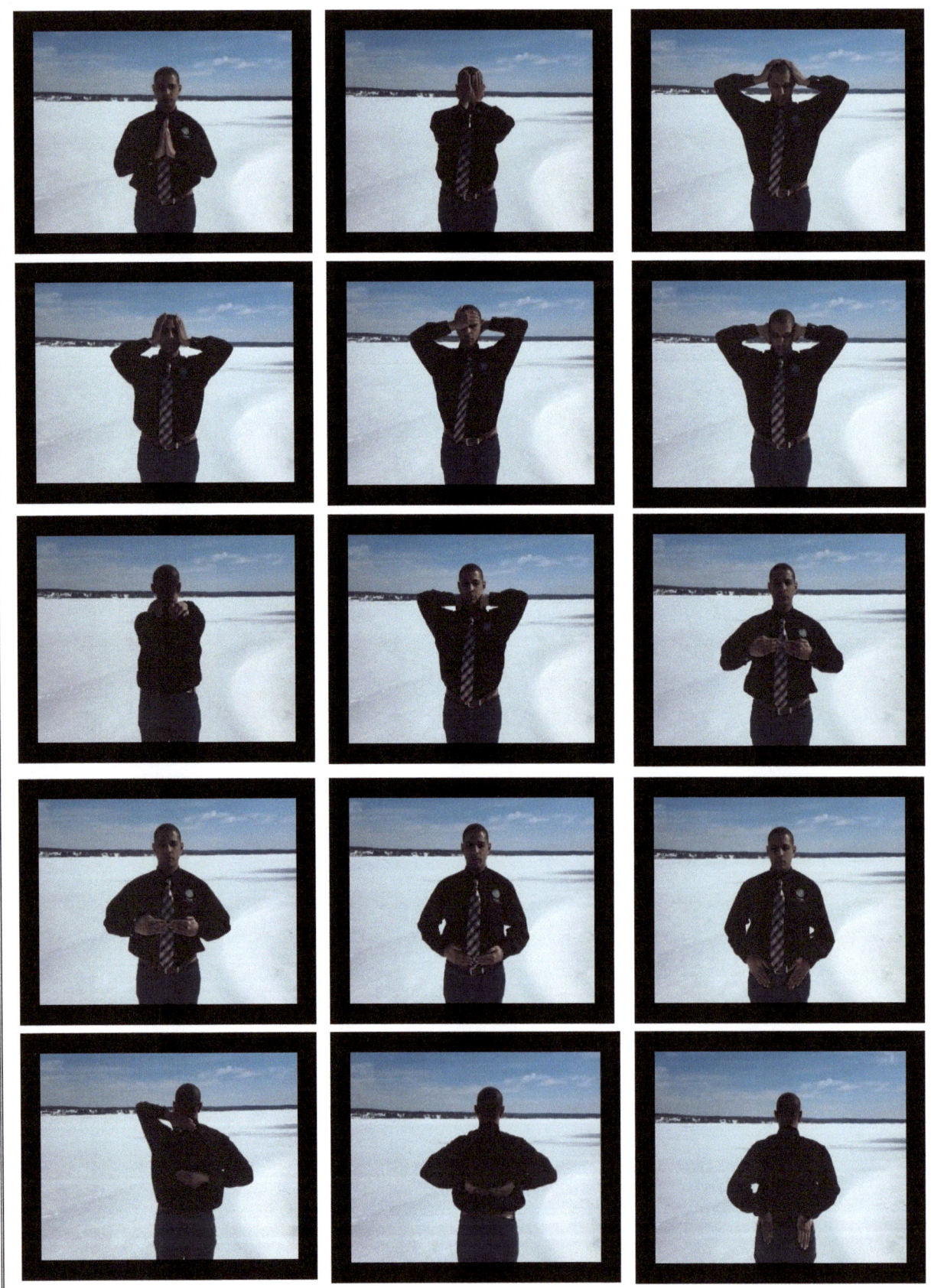

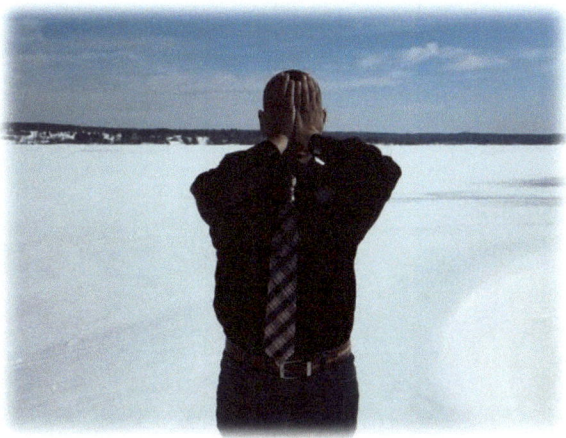

Face

Palms of your hands are placed against your face, cupping your hands over your eyes lightly and fingers upon your forehead. No pressure needed - touch lightly

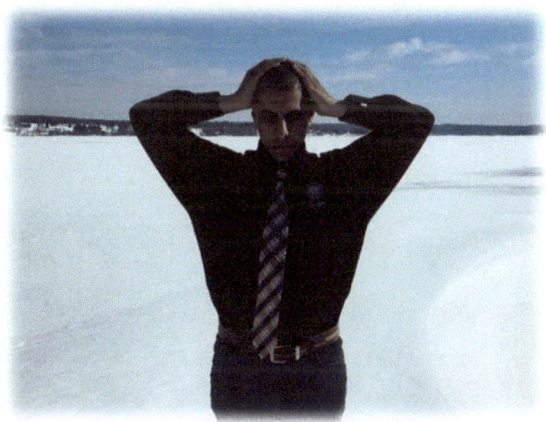

Crown and Top of the Head

Place your hands on both sides of your head, heels of your hands resting near your ears, fingertips touching at the crown.

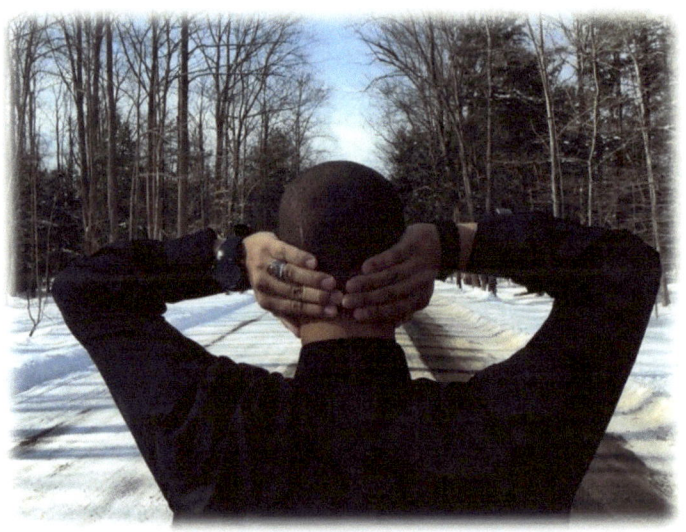

Back of the Head

Crossing your arms behind your head place one hand on the back of your head and the rest the other hand directly above the nape of your neck.

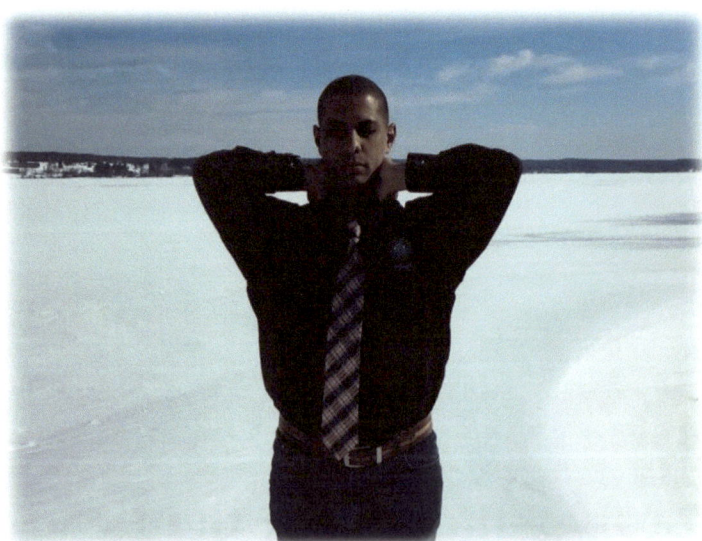

Chin and Jawline

Rest your chin inside the palms of your cupped hands, allow your hands to wrap themselves along your jawline.

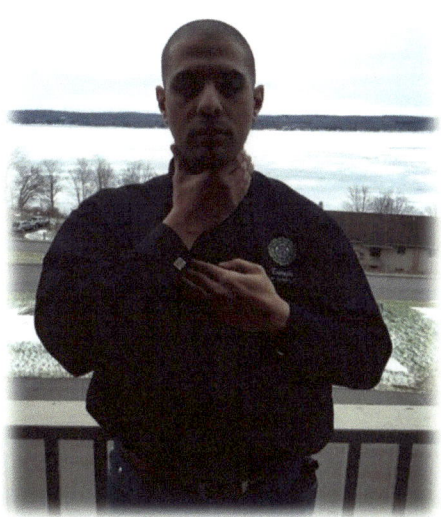

Neck Collarbone and Heart

Grasp your neck comfortably inside the V formed by your thumb and fingers. Lower your other hand and rest it between your collarbone and heart center.

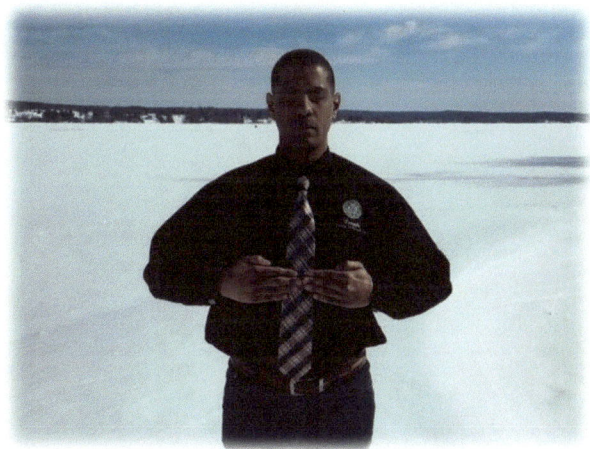

Ribs and Rib Cage

Place your hands on your upper rib cage directly below the breasts. Relax your bent elbows.

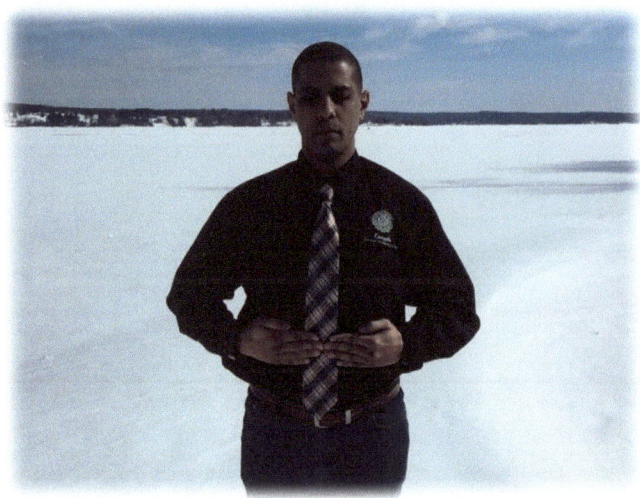

Abdomen

Place your hands on the tummy (solar plexus area) above our navel, allowing your fingertips to touch.

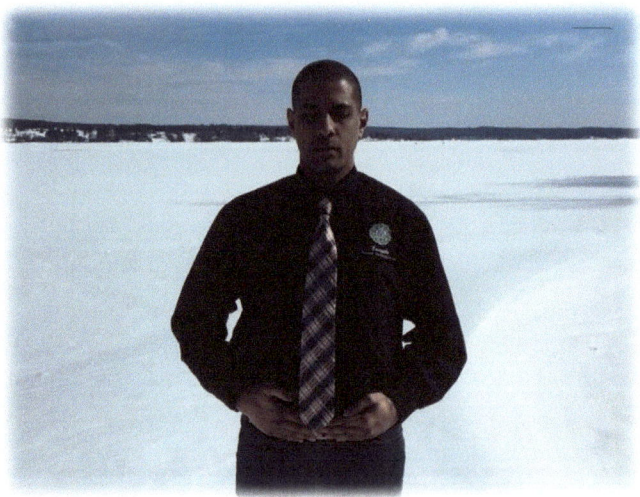

Pelvic Bones

Place one hand over each pelvic bone, again, allowing your fingertips to touch.

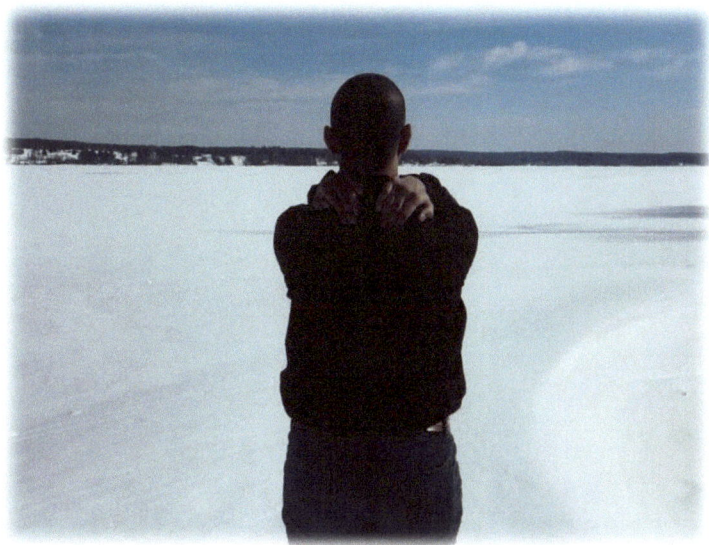

Shoulder Blades

Reach your arms over your head, bending your elbows and placing your hands on your shoulder blades. Alternatively, place your hands on top of your shoulders if you cannot reach your shoulder blades comfortably.

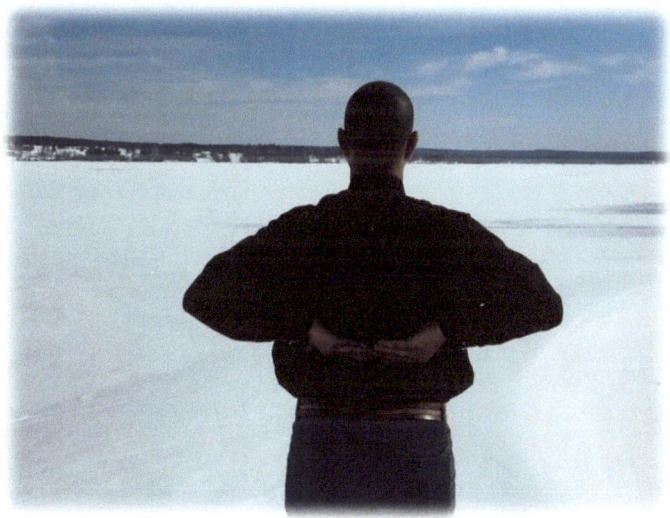

Mid-back

For the mid-back placement, reach behind your back with elbows bent and place your hands on the center of your back.

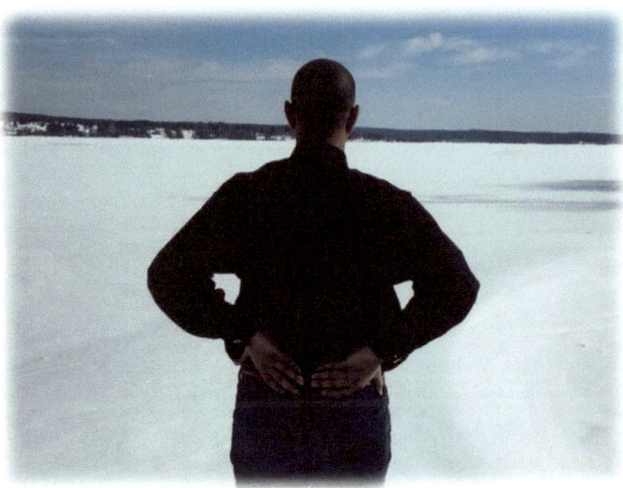

Lower Back

Next hands placements are the on the lower back. Reach behind your back, elbows bent and place your hands on your lower back region.

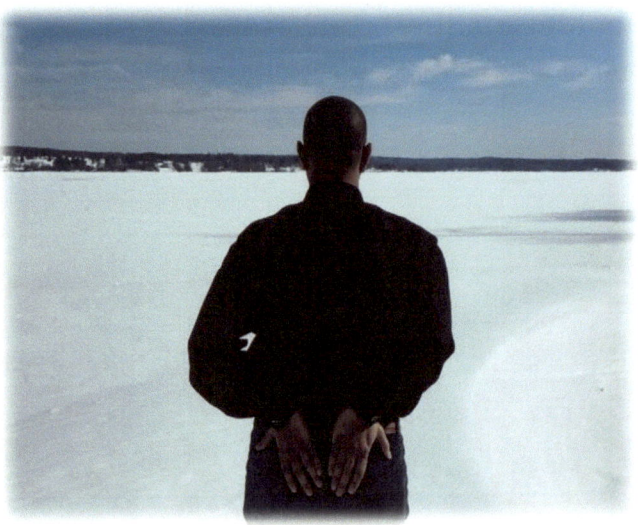

Sacrum

The final hands placement is the sacrum. Lower your arms and place your hands on your sacral region.

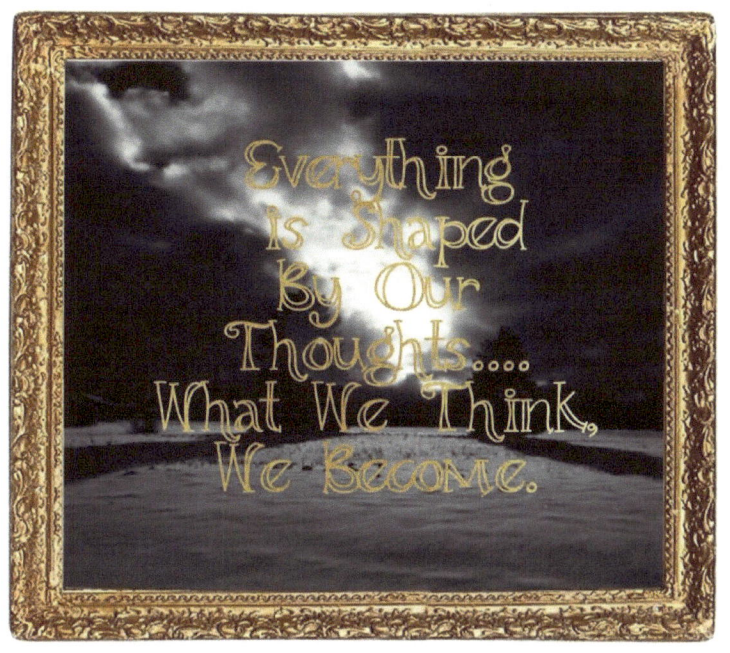

Notes:

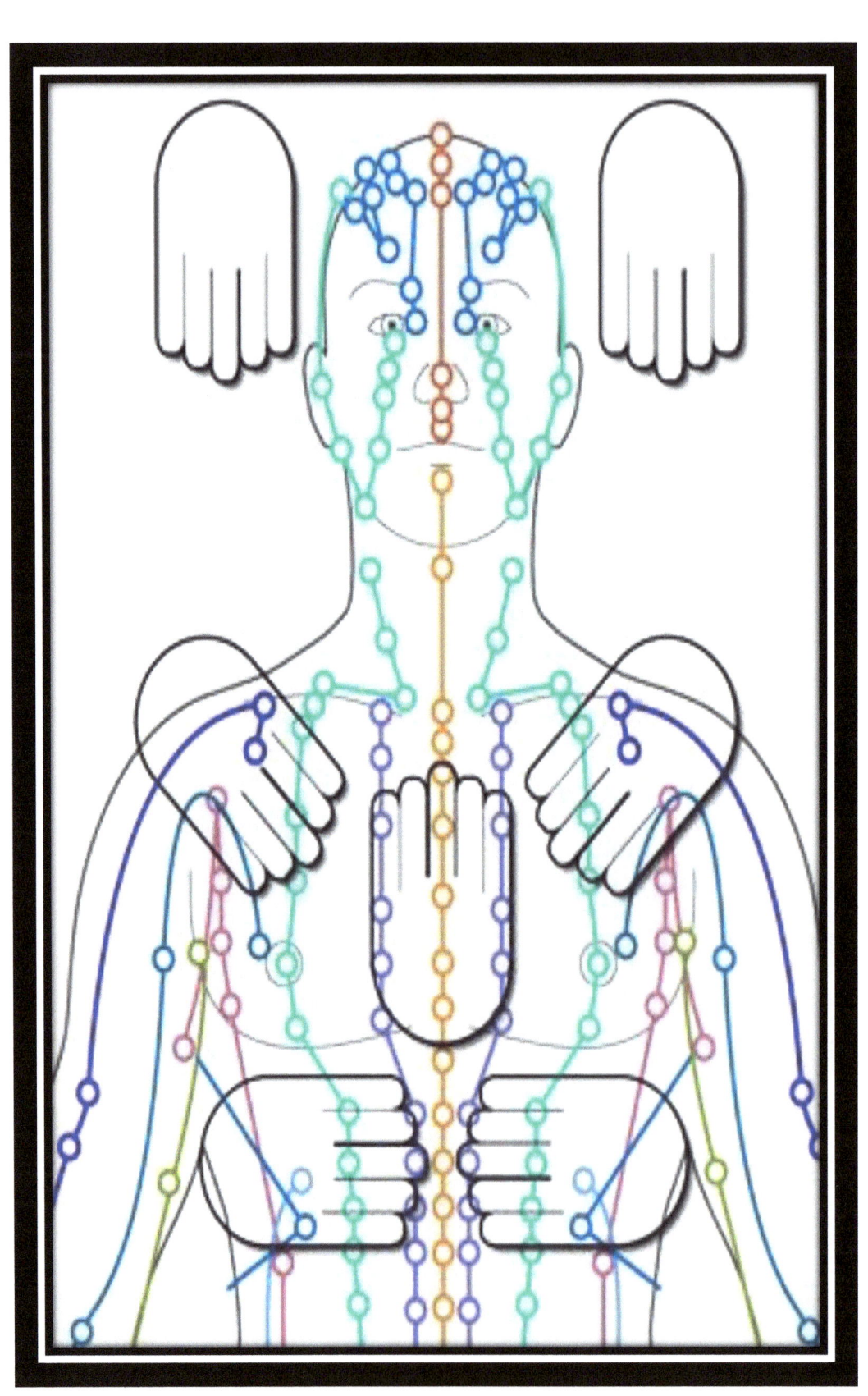

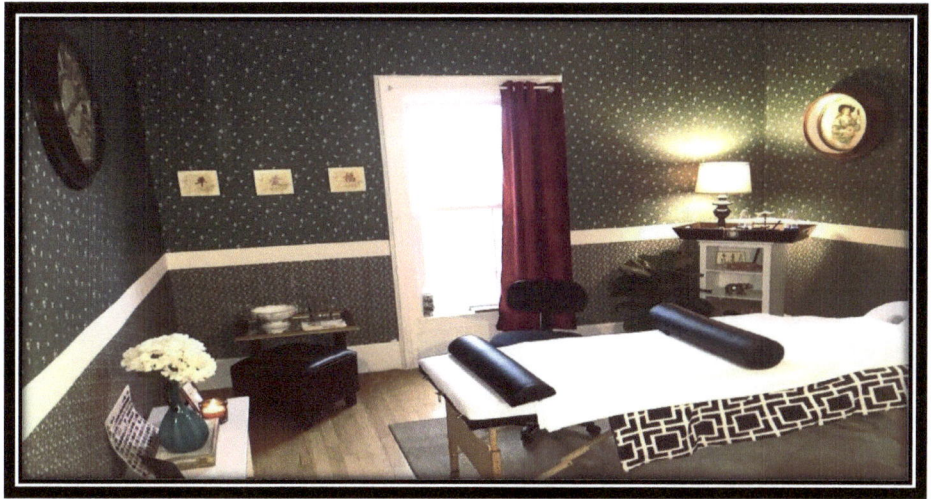

Appropriate Environment

Important to create the right setting whenever possible for reiki healing session.

Work from home or hire a room in a healing center.

The room should be light, clean and feel safe.

Make sure yu will not be interrupted by internal or external distractions.

If you working from home let your family or friends know your schedules so they do not disturb you.

If possible always use a therapy table.

Alternatvely , you could use a strong table with thick blankets on top.

Make sure to be at a comfortable level.

Add a plant to the room and some crystals under the table to help with the right energy.

Some people like to work on total silence.

We prefer to always work with therapeutic music such as classical or ambient or new age to help our clients and ourselves relax.

Burning incense or oils can add a pleasing aroma to you room.

Be carful as some people are sensitive to certain smells and it may cause them to experience an unpleasant therapy session.

Your client may cry as they release blocked emotional issues, so always keep a box of tissue handy.

Remove all jewelry

To enable you work with reiki free from all subtle energy disturbances it is advisable to remove all jewelry such as rings, watches, earrings, chains and necklaces

Remove tight clothing

To allow reiki to flow freely through you and your client it is important that you both remove tight clothing such as belts, ties and shoes

This will also make you feel more comfortable and relaxed

Avoid alcohol

Alcohol dissipates energy

Always refrain from consuming alcohol if you can at least twenty-four hours before a session

Personal hygiene

Ensure you smell and appear clean and fresh

Avoid wearing strong perfume or after shaves

If you smoke make sure you brush your teeth or use a mouth freshener

Refrain from eating food that may leave a smell on your breath

Wash your hands before a reiki session and after

The invocation

It is important to remember that as a reiki practitioner you are not healing your clients

The people receiving reiki are in fact healing themselves

You are merely the channel for reiki

The invocation is a taken that symbolizes you are giving up any claims to power

You are a simply the conduit

Cleanse and harmonize your client aura

Run your hands in your clients' aura 3 times before you begin treatment

Use your intuition sense for possible blockages or hot spots to focus on during your healing session

You are now ready to begin the treatment!!!

Precautions before you give a full treatment reiki session:

- People who has a pacemaker.
- Person who suffers from diabetes mellitus and are taking insulin injections unless they are prepared to check their insulin levels every day as reiki reduces the amount of insulin they require.

Explain to a person who is have their first reiki treatmneyt exactly what you are goingh to do and the type of reactions that moghht occur

Stress that any one of these reactions are normal

Reiki will go wherever it is needed

Beginning The Treatment

Ensure your client is lying flat on the therapy table with their arms down by their sides.

Gently lay your hands on your clients' body. Keep them in each position for between three to five minutes. As you become more experienced use your intuition.

Your hands should be cupped with your fingers firmly closed as though you were trying to hold water.

In the case of burn skin or genitals and breasts hold your hands just above their body.

<u>Notes:</u>

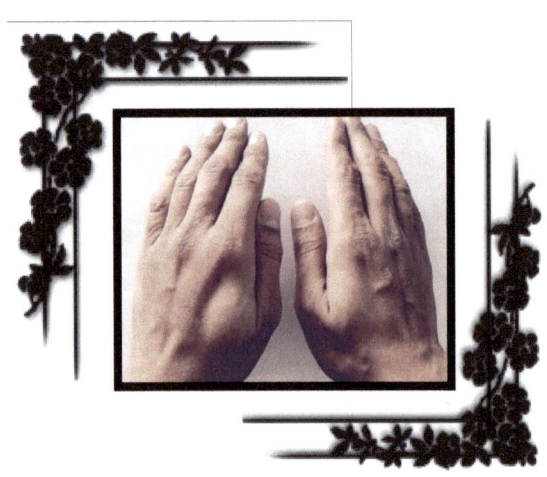

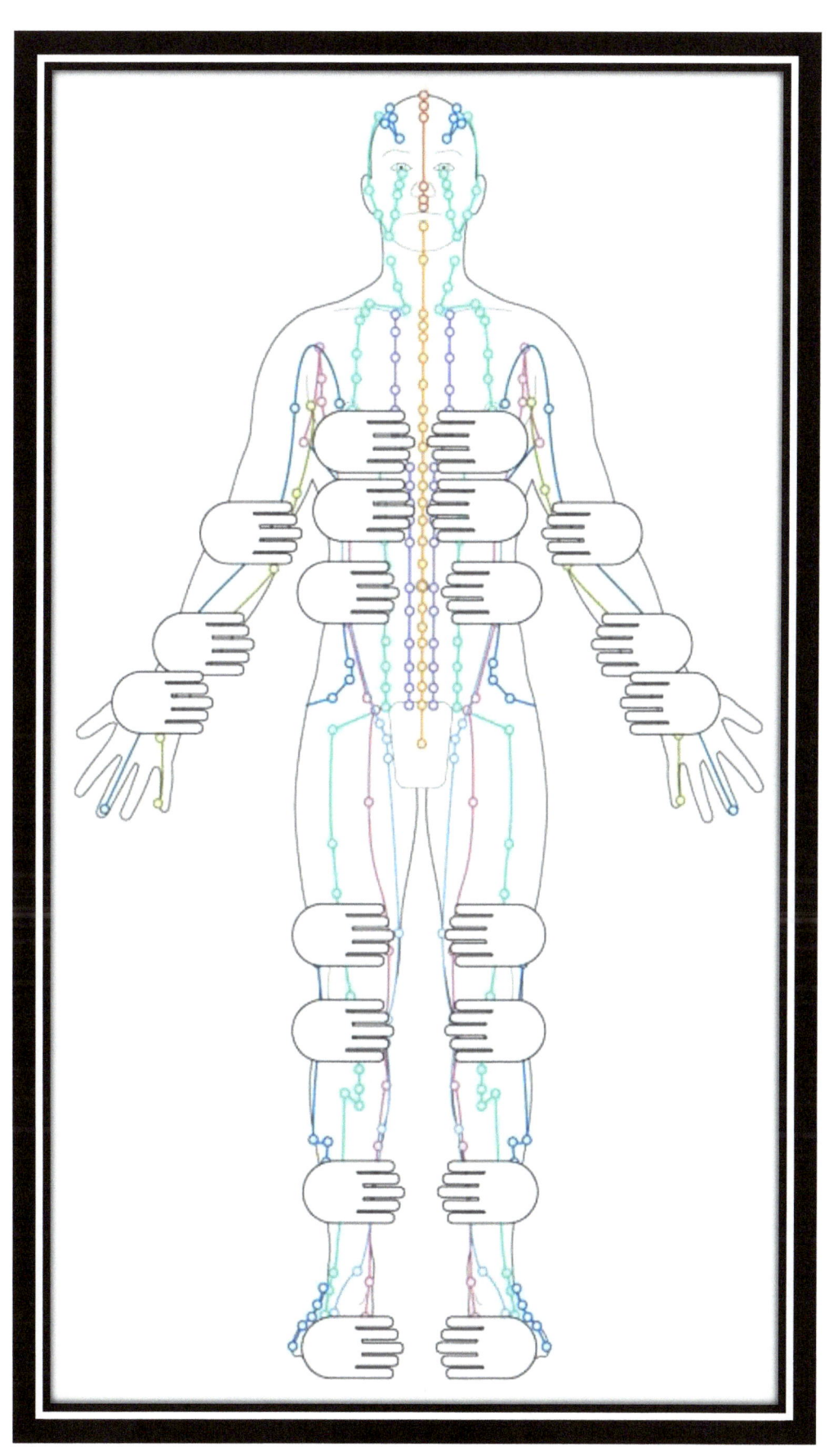

The type of reactions that may occur are:

A sensation of heat

A sensation of cold

See colors

Past life flashes

Involuntary movements

Fall asleep

Itchiness

Emotional responses

Rumbling stomach

Memory flashes

Pins and needles

Sense your hands moving

Often the client will experience extreme cold at the position of your hands while you feel intense heat.

If the client experience nothing explains to them that the reiki energy often works on a subtle level.

Never forget the client is drawing reiki through you, you are the only channel, listen to you clients' body through your hands and treat them as a holistic treatment not symptoms.

Sense the different types of energy, use your intuition.

A full body treatment takes 60-90 minutes at the end of a treatment always offer your client a glass of cold water to aid grounding always wash your hands under cold running water after each treatment.

When all the positions have been treated place your left hand on the client crown chakra and your right hand at the base of their spine this final position balances the energy in your clients' body.

Complete your treatment by combing your clients' aura 3 times.

First: firm stroke on body

Second: light stroke on body

Third: in aura above body

Each time touching the floor to ground your client.

"Believe Creates the Actual Fact."

- William James

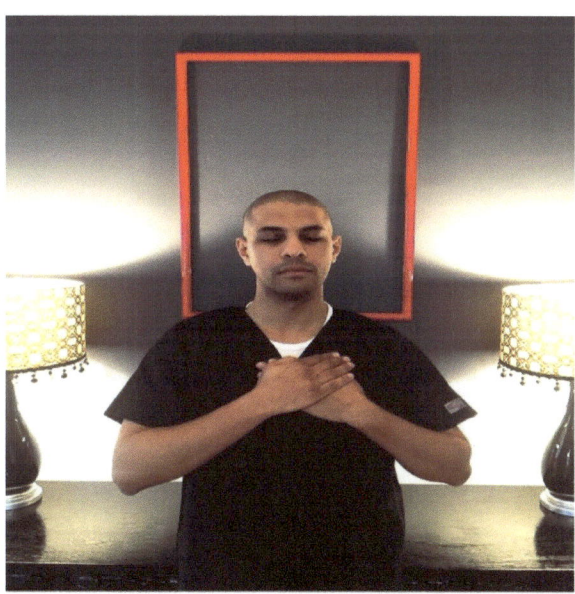

Chapter 17: Using Reiki with patients

Reiki in the Clinical Setting

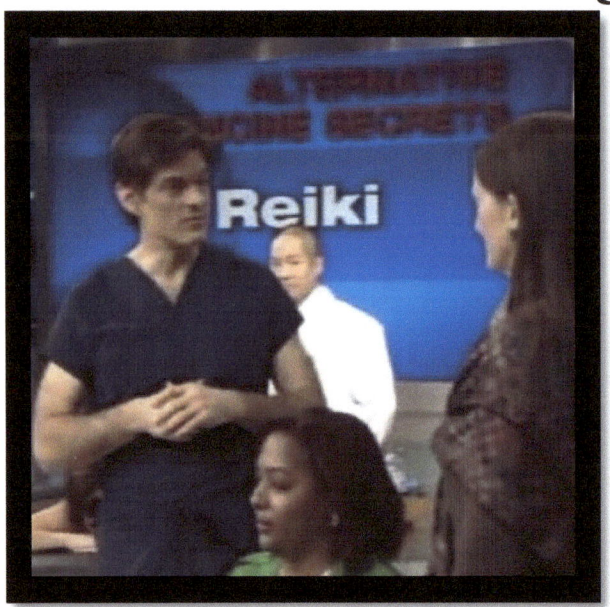

Reiki in the Clinical Setting is On The Rise

Reiki is increasingly finding its way into institutional settings, from hospitals to hospices, and the push appears to be coming from patients as well as clinical practitioners.

"More and more, patients are requesting care beyond what most consider to be traditional health services, and hospitals are responding to the needs of the communities they serve by offering these therapies," according to researcher Sita Ananth of Health Forum, an affiliate of the American Hospital Association (AHA). "And hospitals are responding to the needs of the communities they serve by offering these therapies."

Dr. Oz used Reiki in His Practice for Over 10 Years

Dr. Oz has conducted research on the effects of Reiki on his surgical patients with Julie Motz, RN, a Reiki-trained therapist, who assisted Dr. Oz during 11 open heart surgeries and heart transplants. These 11 patients had no post-operative depression, pain or leg weakness; no organ rejection (in transplants); a better functioning immune system, and a positive attitude toward healing.

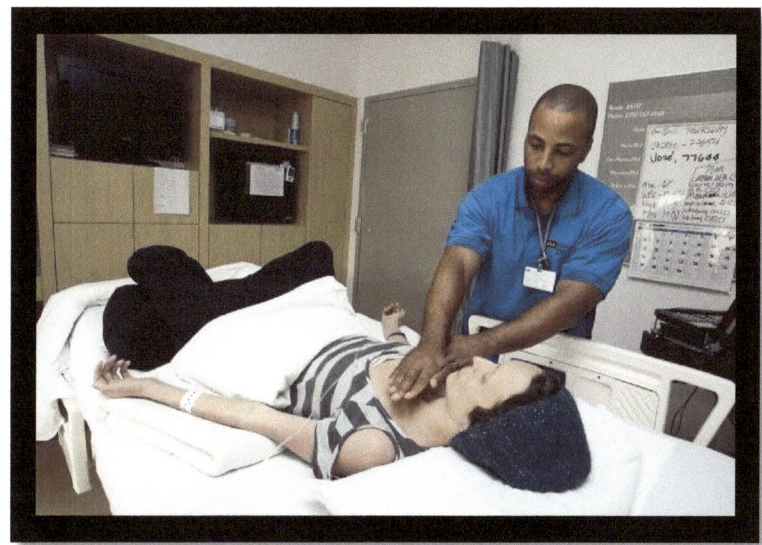

Reiki is now one of the top three complementary in-patient therapies in U.S. hospitals, according to an AHA survey. Massage therapy takes first place, with 37% of hospital patients requesting it. Number two is music and art therapy at 25%, and a very close third is "healing touch therapies" at 25%, which included Reiki and Therapeutic Touch.

Hospitals are responding, discovering for themselves the many benefits Reiki can offer. "As our health care system challenges institutions to offer high-quality but cost-effective service, Reiki is being recognized as an important tool to maximize patient care and minimize recovery time," according to Libby Barnett and Maggie Babb, co-authors of *Reiki Energy Medicine: Bringing Healing Touch into Home, Hospital and Hospice.*

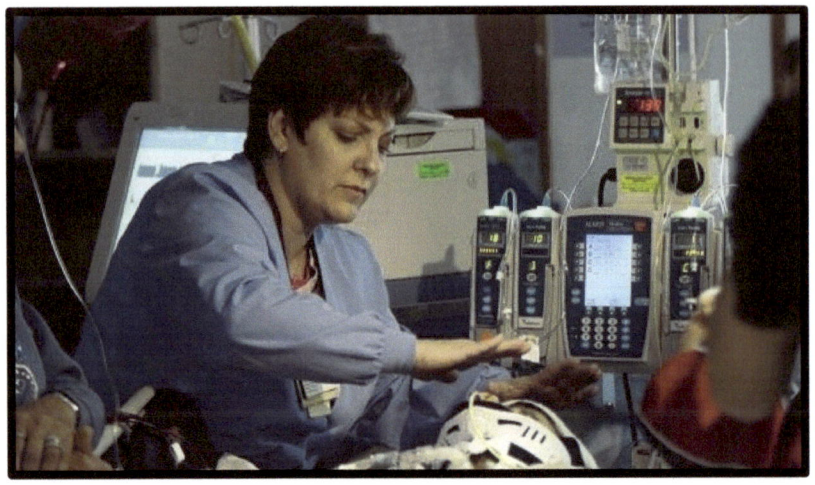

An Emerging Role in Health Care

Reiki has become recognized as a valuable source of pain management and symptom relief in hospice and palliative care. Some mainstream medical organizations include it as a component of wellness or pain management. Reiki also can be used during invasive procedures, chemotherapy, or even surgery. Certain hospital oncology departments and cancer wellness centers are informing clients about Reiki, and many even include Reiki practitioners as part of their teams.

Dr. Susan Pocotte, a nurse researcher studying the use of Reiki in rehabilitation settings, notes that the "holistic approach to nursing is congruous with integrating Reiki into nursing care.... Hospitals and clinics use three different methods of Reiki delivery: licensed professionals such as nurses, Reiki practitioners, and education programs to train patients, family members, and caregivers in first-degree Reiki."

What Nurses and Physicians say about Reiki in the Clinical Setting?

Mounting anecdotal evidence confirms its benefits over and over again. Nurses and physicians who use Reiki in the clinical setting consistently say it: Makes a patient relaxed, calm and cooperative; relieves acute and chronic pain; boosts the immune system; reduces stress; decreases the need for pain medication; improves sleep and appetite; accelerates the healing process; and has no side effects or contraindications. They also say that Reiki reduces many of the unwanted side effects of radiation and chemotherapy, including nausea and fatigue.

Ongoing Research- Reiki and Surgery

Perhaps most importantly, increasing research allows Western healthcare practitioners to see quantifiable data about the effects of Reiki on patients with a variety of conditions. The largest ongoing study of Reiki in the clinical setting continues to be conducted at Columbia/HCA Portsmouth Regional Hospital, Portsmouth, NH, where more than 8,000 surgical patients have been given pre- and post-surgery Reiki treatments. Reiki is incorporated into their admission procedure and is also administered during transport to surgery. Treatments are given by trained RNs, physical therapists, technicians and support staff.

Research results continue to be consistent. All the patients in this study who received Reiki had the need for less anesthesia, had less bleeding during surgery, used less pain medications, had shorter lengths of stay in the hospital, and indicated greater satisfaction with their hospital experience than other patients.

Reiki for Pain Management

The Cross Cancer Institute in Edmonton, Canada, conducted a study on the effects of Reiki with 20 oncology patients in chronic pain. Study supervisors used both a VAS (visual analog scale) and Likert scale to measure pain before and after Reiki, and their conclusion was that Reiki greatly improved pain levels.

Reiki and Oncology

Other research with oncology patients shows that Reiki speeds up the elimination of toxins, improves immune response, helps manage side effects of chemotherapy and radiation, and helps reduce the inevitable fear and anxiety that accompanies a cancer diagnosis.

Reiki and the Heart

The Section of Cardiology, Department of Internal Medicine, at Yale University conducted a study to determine if Reiki would improve Heart Rate

Variability (HRV) in patients recovering from acute coronary syndrome. Reiki is an ongoing clinical program offered on Yale-New Haven Hospital cardiac units, so the Reiki therapists in this study were 5 Reiki-trained nurses already employed in that program. To compare Reiki to musical intervention and resting control, continuous electrocardiographic readings were obtained for 12 control, 13 music, and 12 Reiki patients. The change with Reiki was significantly greater than with music (p=0.007) or resting (p=0.025).

Reiki and Chronic Illnesses

Several studies on Reiki and chronic illness indicate improvement in spleen, lymphatic and nervous system function in patients with multiple sclerosis, lupus, fibromyalgia and thyroid disorder, as well as better management of symptoms in patients with AIDS, chronic fatigue syndrome, and sleep disorders.

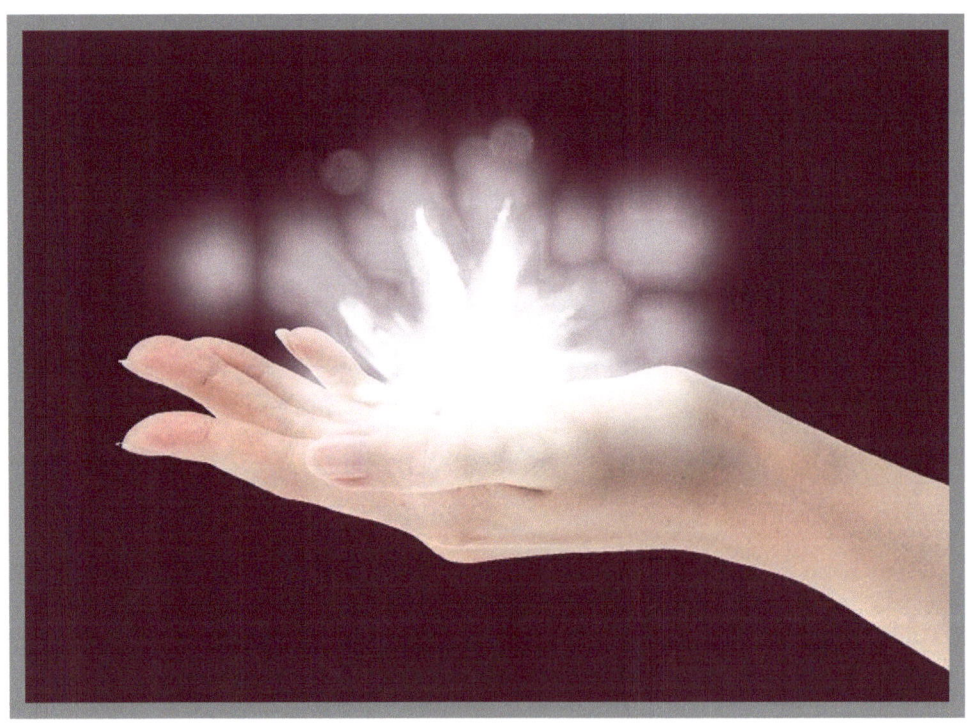

Chapter 18: Rapid Reiki Session

(When time is limited you can perform a shortened Reiki session that is still quite effective. Please note there is a hand-out in the supplementary materials section. This hand-out includes the root chakra position in case you feel you want to include it in some of your sessions)

It is not always possible to spend 60-90 minutes conducting a reiki treatment, often the person requiring reiki has a limited time.

There is quick alternative for these situations, a rapid reiki treatment focuses on the chakra points while the client sits in a chair and takes about 15-30 minutes

Position No. 1: Stand behind your client

Stand behind the client with your hands on their shoulders

(remember your invocations)

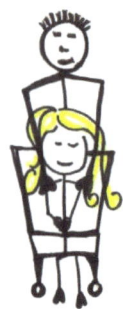

Position No. 2: Remain behind your client

Place both of your hands on their crown chakra.

Position No.2

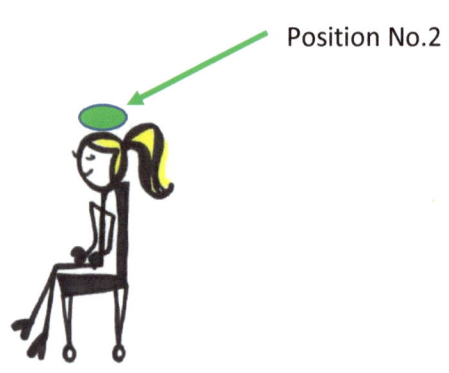

Position No. 3: Move to the side of your client

Place one hand on the 3rd eye and one hand on the occipital ridge.

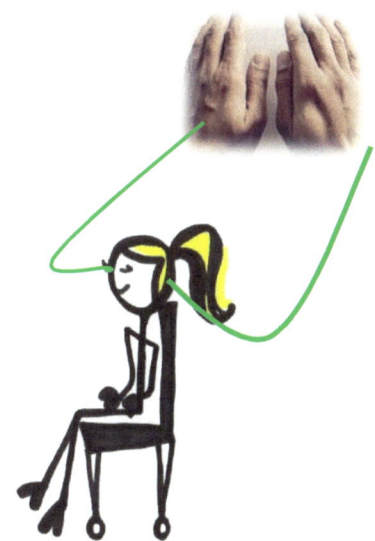

Position No. 4: Remain at the side of your client

Place one hand on the throat chakra & one hand at the back of your client's neck.

Position No. 5: Remain at the side of your client

Place one hand on the solar plexus chakra & one hand at the back of their spine.

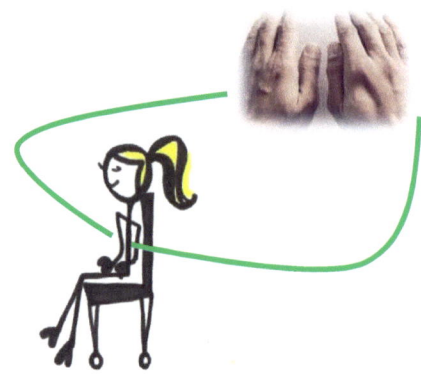

Position No. 6: Remain at the side of your client

Place one hand on the sacral chakra & the other hand on the back of their spine.

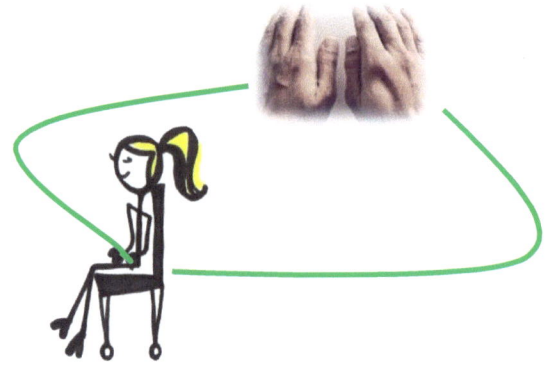

Position No. 7: Move to the front of your client

Place one hand on each of your clients knees.

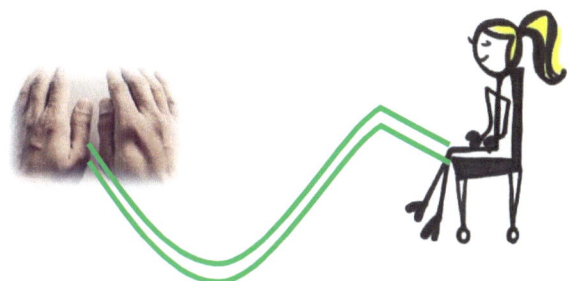

Position No. 8: Kneel Down in Front of your client

Place one hand on each of your client's feet.

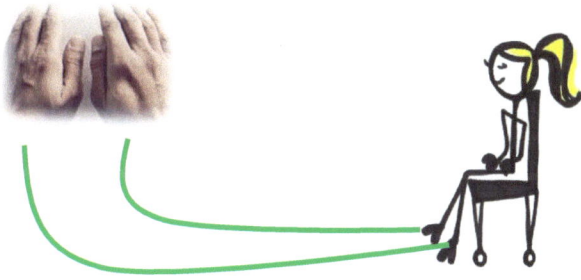

Finally comb your clients aura 3 times as you normally would after a full treatment.

Wash your hands in cold running water and offer a cold drink to your client to assist in grounding them.

Chapter 19: Reiki Group Session

(Learn how to perform a Reiki session with other practitioners)

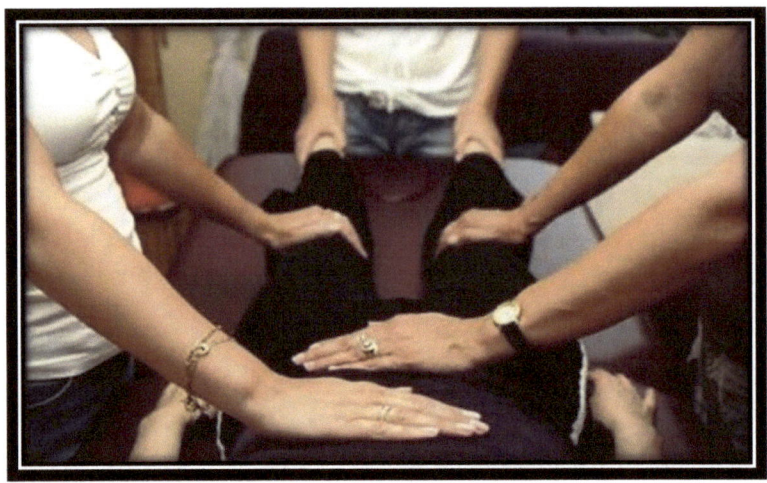

Group treatments were first used by Dr. Hayashi at his clinic in Tokyo

He would often treat clients with the help of several other reiki practitioners.

The befits of group treatment:

Group treatment is quicker taking as little as 6-10 minutes to complete a full reiki treatment

Very powerful the client receives an intense healing energy

Allows the team to form a bond and create a unique energy

Client will often notice the different energy vibrations from different reiki practitioners

Guidelines for a group treatment:

Normal preparation

Before you begin a group treatment decide who will work on the head positions and ultimately control the healing session

Decide who will complete the session by smoothing the clients' aura.

You can have one practitioner at each end of the clients' body while the other practitioners work in the middle

Don't forget tissue

A wondeful way to treat many people quickly an dideal for therapy day

Remember to wash your hands before and after each treatment under cold running water to didipate any negatibve energy and assist grounding for each member of the team

Spend time sharing experinces. Group treatment is a great way to learn and grow toghether.

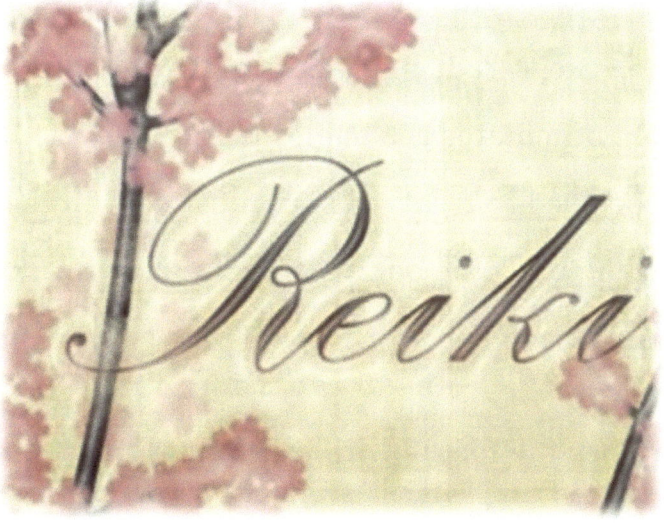

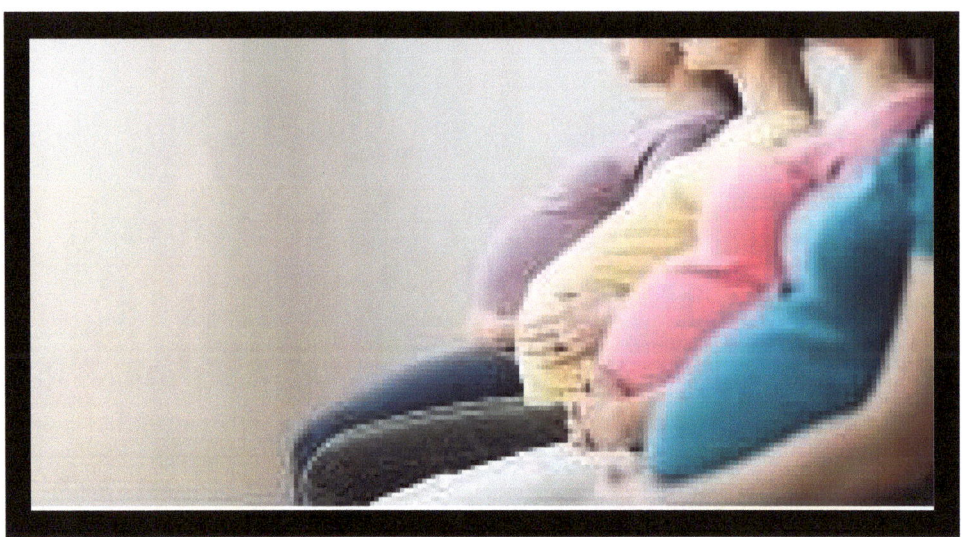

Chapter 20: Pregnancy, Babies & Children

(Reiki is a safe and effective way to work with women during their pregnancy as well as with babies and children)

Pregnancy

Reiki is both safe and extremely beneficial to an unborn child and their pregnant mother

Reiki can help during pregnancy in so many ways icluding :

Reiki alleviations morning sickness

Reiki reducing stress and tiredness

Reiki stimulates the babies healthy development

Reiki can be used to treat painful muscles, joints or the spine

Reiki strenghtens the bond btween a mother and her baby

Reiki keeps the mind body and spirit in balance reducing the chances of post natal deprssion

Reiki nourishes the foetus with love and the universla life force

If the father is a reiki practitioner he can slao help during the pregnancy by treating his partner.

The important bond between father and child will also be stimulated.

Reiki can help couples who are finding it difficult to conceive by reducing stress and stimulating both the females natural reproductive cycle and the males' production of sperm.

Babies:

Reiki can accelerate the recovery time of mother and baby after birth.

Reiki can be used to heal the babies umbilical cord.

Reiki can be used to vitalized and nourish the mother's milk or baby formula.

Nourished and satisfy babies sleep better. Something all parents pray for.

Reiki stimulates balance in the new born baby.

Reiki can be used to help treat cradle cap, colic and wind.

Important Note:

Always consult your doctor no matter how trivial it may seem if you are concerned about your baby.

Children:

Reiki can be used to treat your children throughout their lives

Reiki is wonderful for all their aches and pains.

Reiki is a special gift you can share with your children.

Children love reiki!

Use reiki at bedtime to help your children drift off to sleep.

Reiki balance your child's mind body and spirit leading to a clearer more focused approach to life.

Chapter 21: Reiki and Palliative Care (Reiki and Death)

(Reiki can also be used in cases of terminal illness to help an individual and their loved ones process the transition)

Reiki and End of Life Issues

For end of life issues, hospice studies show that Reiki addresses physical and emotional symptoms while improving quality of life during palliative care. Reiki promotes deep relaxation, pain management, and relief from depression with less medication. It also facilitates release of anxiety, grief and fear, supporting positive emotional closure with loved ones and a calm, peaceful passing.

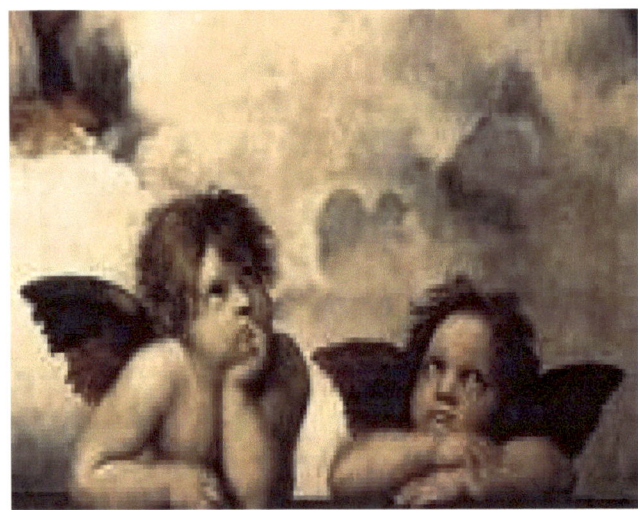

When a person become more spiritually aware they grow to understand and accept these ancient beliefs.

Use reiki with a person who is terminally ill, connect them to the unconditional love of God & prepare them for their transition. Reiki can revitalize them. Working with people who are dying connects us to the universal life force. Death is not failure it is a natural part of life.

Chapter 22: Reiki Treatment: Animals and Nature

(Learn how to perform a Reiki session with Animals and plants)

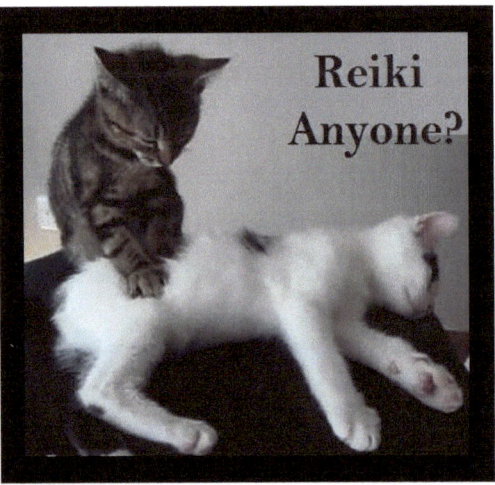

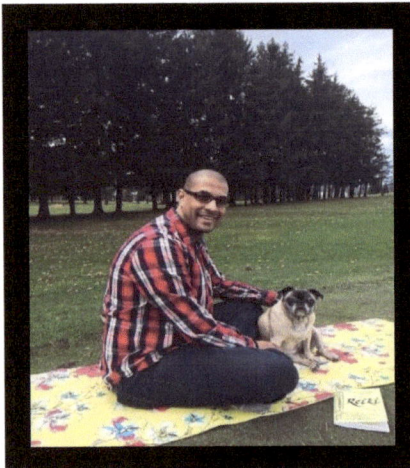

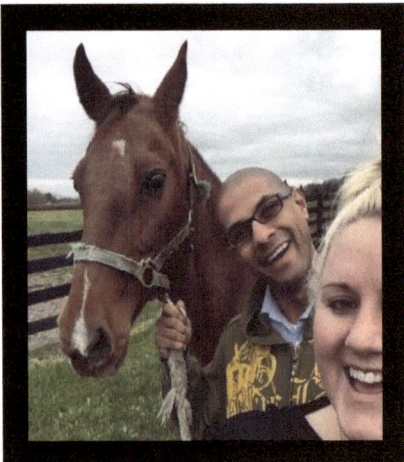

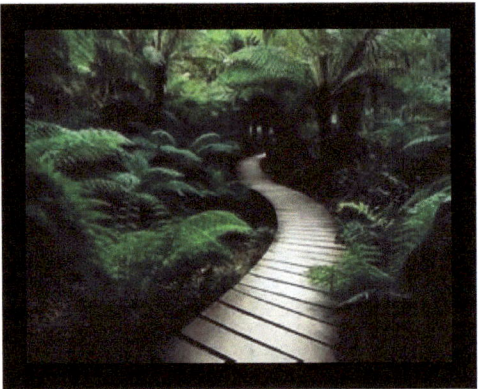

Basic techniques for animals:

Simply cup hands around small animal or bird, for larger animals such as cats, dogs, horses etc. by placing your hands behind their ears & work around their body as with a normal full treatment for humans.

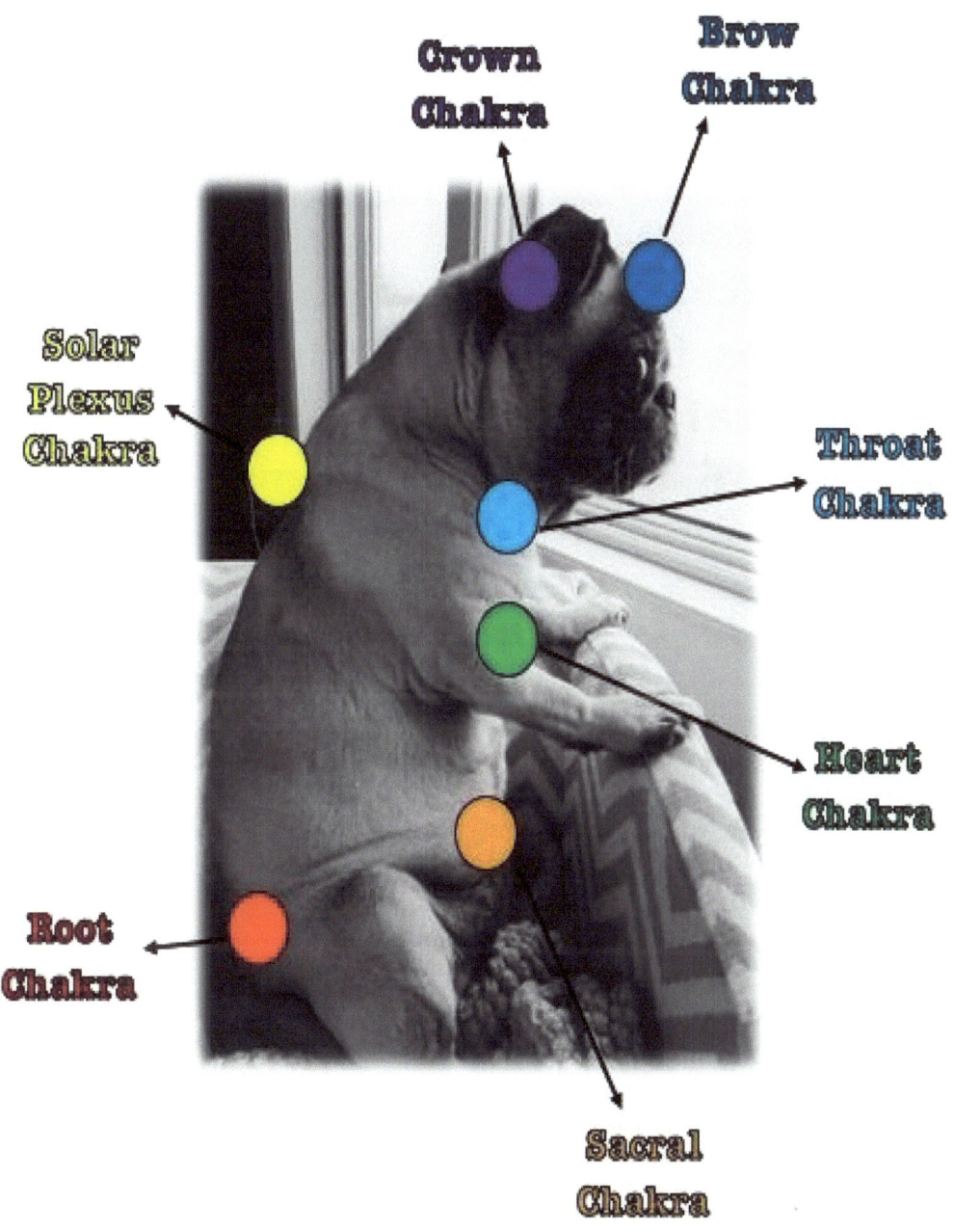

Section Three Quiz:

1. What is Reiki Attunement?

2. What should you do after you have been attuned for level I?

3. What is the number of hand treatments usually used to treat yourself and others?

4. Before and after a Reiki treatment to another person you should do what?

5. What is Gassho?

6. When completing a client session, how many times is it best to run through your client's aura?

7. What health precautions should you know before completing a treatment to a client?

8. What is a rapid Reiki session?

9. True/False, Reiki is good to use on a pregnant woman, babies and those in hospice?

10. True/False, Reiki can be used on all living things?

Answers: #1 The Reiki first degree attunements connect you to the Reiki source and allow healing energy to flow through you. The attunements are passed by a Reiki Master in a sacred ceremony that connects upper chakras and the palms of the hands to the Reiki source using sacred Reiki symbols. #2. For Three weeks meditate every day and give yourself a self-healing. #3. There are several but 22 are the main hand treatments. #4. Cleanse your hands and your patients' hands with water to disconnect the energy. #5. Gassho means 'hands together', and the correct position is to have your hands together in front of your chest (like praying hands), just above your heart, so that you can breathe out onto your fingertips. Hold this position for meditation. #6. You should run through the Aura three times. #7. Check health precautions for those who use a pacemaker. Persons who suffer from diabetes mellitus and are taking insulin injections unless they are prepared to check their insulin levels every day as reiki reduces the amount of insulin they require. #9. True, Reiki works amazingly for woman, babies and those in hospice. #10. True, Reiki works on all living things. All living things use energy vibrations.

Section 5: Reiki I Conclusion

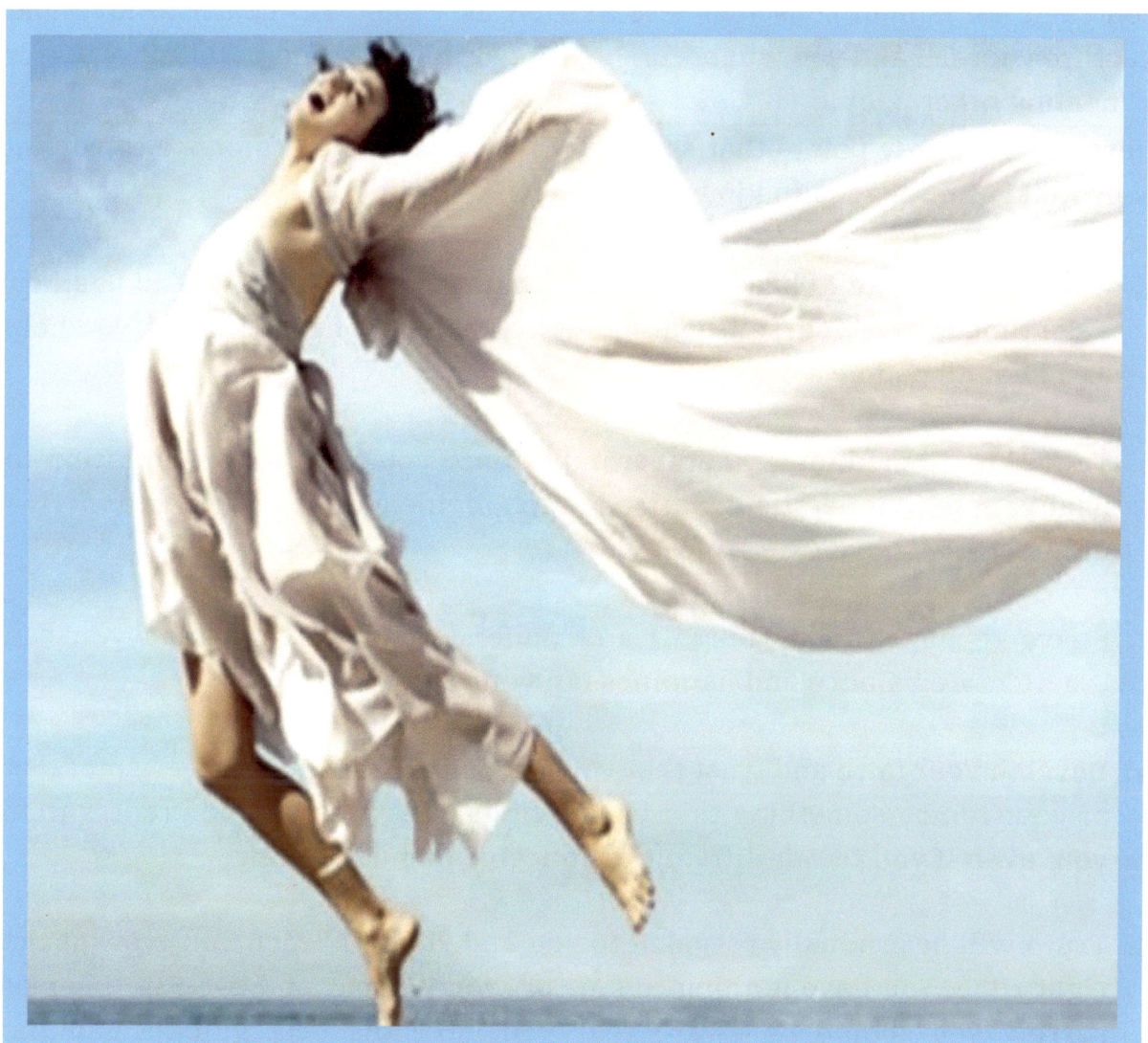

Chapter 24: Reiki Level I Conclusion

(This section concludes the First degree of Usui Reiki)

By undertaking your own path of self-healing you are helping yourself and other people of this world. Through your own personal and spiritual growth, you raise all human consciousness as well as your own. Learn to love and nurture yourself and you will become stronger, happier and potentially better at healing other people.

Here are some key points that summarize my advice and guidance to you on your Reiki and self-healing journey:

1. Trust that as a Reiki healer you are a channel for divine love and healing. Take time to give yourself-healing. As you help and heal yourself, you help and heal all people

2. Take time to meditate, whatever experience you have. Use meditation to heal yourself, understand yourself, seek divine guidance or create divine union

3. Strive to understand yourself and understand ways in which you can create more balance and happiness in your life.

4. Develop your faith and trust that you are helped and guided every moment of your life by something that is conscious, wise, loving and greater than you, even if you find it difficult to conceive of such a thing.

5. Truth will be gradually revealed to you and you will learn and grow at the right time. You have nothing to fear or worry about and even in times of sorrow you should be aware that you have the best guidance in the universe at your side, giving you help, love and healing.

6. Reiki 1 beginning of a wonderful journey. Embrace Reiki into your daily healthcare practice that will helps to accelerate the natural healing process. Reiki works seamlessly with other disciplines and healing modalities.

7. Continue to study Reiki II – A certified Reiki Practitioner level II

and Reiki Master – A certified Reiki Master Teacher level III

8. It is a privilege to be your Reiki Teacher, thank you! I endeavor to help you in your self - healing and your Reiki healing and I am always willing to give help, guidance, advice and healing to you.

Increase your abilities and skills of healing by continue education and study one or more of our coming courses and workshops; Recommended for you:

- Reiki for Animals
- Psychic Surgery
- Reiki for Children
- Chakra balance
- Kundalini power
- Reiki for Her (prenatal, Pregnancy, post-natal & babies)
- Reiki for relationships
- Grounding
- Connecting heaven with earth
- Reiki in Nursing school
- Reiki in Medical school
- Reiki Anatomy
- Reiki ethics, professional bodies and standard of practice
- Establish your reiki business practice
- Reiki evidence base studies
- Reiki and the Globe
- Reiki hand positions and treatment
- Reiki and depression
- Reiki and the five elements
- (focus, sleep better, less stress, more energy, relax)
- Reiki Hands and Acu-points

The learning journey is endless and investment in yourself is the best in life!

Congratulations On Completing Reiki Level I- Reiki Practitioner!

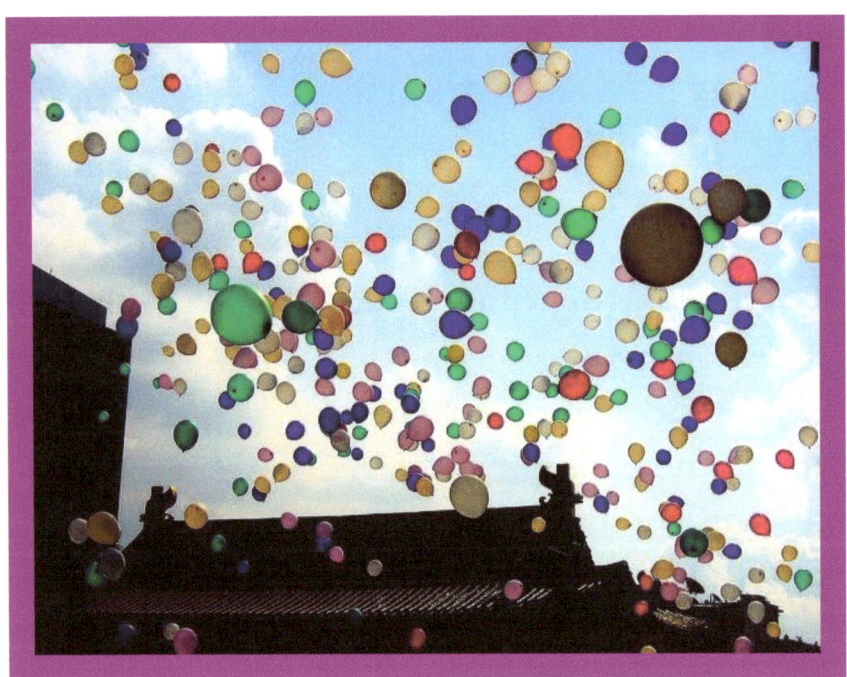

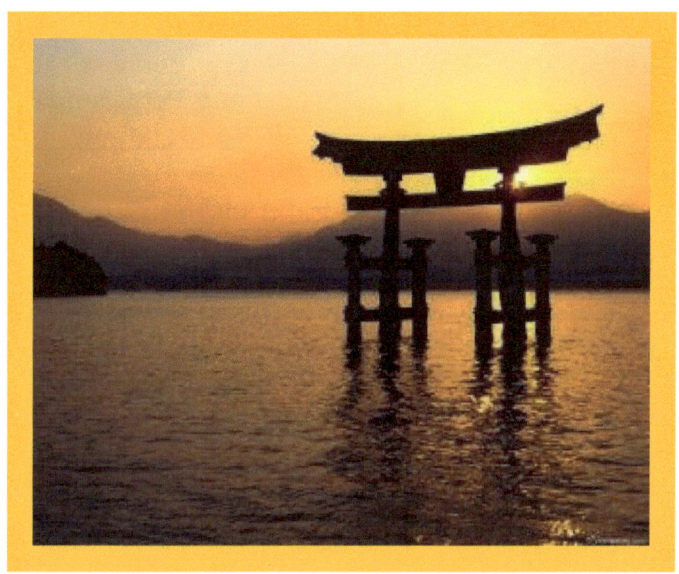

Section 5: Appendix

References and Further Reading

Alandydy, Patricia, BSN, RN. **"Using Reiki to Support Surgical Patients."** Journal of Nursing Care Quality, April 1999, Vol.13, No. 4, pp. 89-91.

Barnett, Libby and Babb, Maggie, **"Reiki Energy Medicine: Bringing Healing Touch into Home, Hospital and Hospice,"** Healing Arts Press.

Bossi, RN, MS, CS, Larraine; DeCristofaro, RN, MS, OCN, and Ott, RN, MN, MEd, CS, Mary Jane. **"Reiki Treatments for People Living with Cancer."** Virginia Henderson International Nursing Library.

Bossi, RN, MS, CS, Larraine; DeCristofaro, RN, MS, OCN, and Ott, RN, MN, MEd, CS, Mary Jane. **"Reiki as a Clinical Intervention in Oncology Nursing Practice."** Clinical Journal of Oncology Nursing, Vol. 12, No. 3/2008, pp. 489-494.

Brewitt, B., Vittetoe, T, and Hartwell, B. **"The Efficacy of Reiki Hands-On Healing: Improvements in Spleen and Nervous System Function as Quantified by Electro-Dermal Screening."** Alternative Therapies, July 1997, Vol.3, No.4, pg.89

Olson, Karin, R.N., Ph.D., and John Hanson, MSc. **"Using Reiki to Manage Pain: a Preliminary Report."** Cancer Prevention and Control, June 1997, Vol.1, No. 2, pages 108-13.

Singg, Sangreeta and Linda J. Dressen. **"Desirable Self-Perceived Psychophysiological Changes in Chronically Ill Patients: An Experiential Study of Reiki."** International Society for the Study of Subtle Energy and Energy Medicine, June 1999.

Wardell, Diane Wind and Joan Engebretson, **"Biological Correlates of Reiki Touch™ Healing,"** Journal of Advanced Nursing, Feb. 2001, Vol. 33, No. 4: pp. 439-445.

Rachel S.C. Friedman, MD, Matthew M. Burg, PhD, Pamela Miles, BA, Forrester Lee, MD and Rachel Lampert, MD, **"Effects of Reiki on Autonomic Activity Early After Acute Coronary**

Syndrome," Section of Cardiology, Department of Internal Medicine, Yale University, School of Medicine, 333 Cedar Street, FMP 3, New Haven, Connecticut 06520

Dekel, Natalie and Gil. (2008) **Introduction to Reiki and Personal Development.** http://www.poeticmind.co.uk/wellbeing/introduction-to-reiki-and-personal-development/

Tamisha, Sabrina. (2003) **The Science Behind Reiki - What Happens in a Treatment?** UK Reiki Federation. http://www.reikifed.co.uk/index.htm [Accessed 18 November, 2003]

The Original Reiki Handbook of Dr. Mikao Usui
Frank Arjava Petter and Mikao Usui, Lotus Press, Shangri-La

http://www.americannursetoday.com/reiki-ancient-healing-art-for-todays-new-healthcare-vision/

Reiki Hand positions by, Kiyoshi Takahashi: http://www.reikitechnician.com/

Google Scholar-General Research & Articles

Photos- Bing.com (approved commercial use)

IRAP- International Reiki Association Professionals

Reiki Code of Ethics and Standards of Practice

It is only a qualified and registered medical practitioner who is allowed to diagnose medical conditions. Reiki practitioners are not allowed to make any diagnosis or claim to be able to cure any condition. A responsible Reiki practitioner should ensure that clients seek proper medical treatment and that animals have been seen by a vet. Furthermore, clients should let their doctor know that they are receiving Reiki treatment.

Reiki Insurance

Before treating someone professionally it is advisable to be insured for professional malpractice and for public liability. This insurance is not too expensive but does have some requirements of practitioners, such as keeping client records. Our practice and my work is insured policy #: PHPK1443616-000

Professional Bodies and Regulation of Practice

There are many Reiki professional bodies that support their members in the USA, Such as The International Association of Reiki Professional (IARP). Registered as a Reiki Master Practitioner/Teacher Member ID 28895077

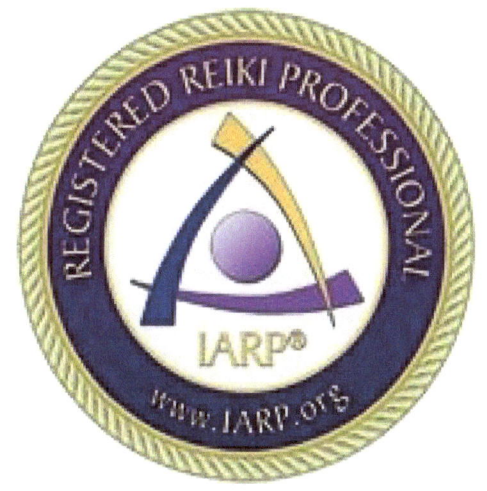

Help and Support

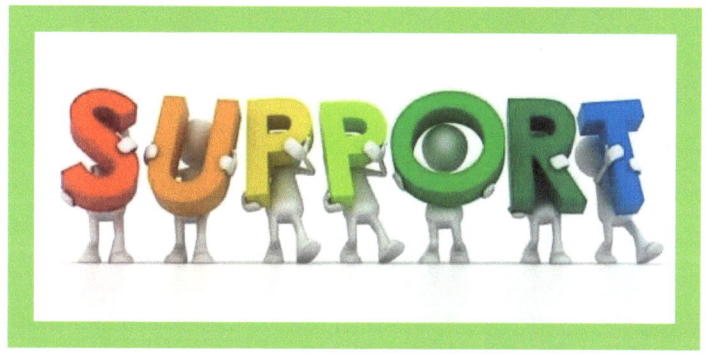

It is my great honor to be your Reiki Master Teacher. I am committed to giving you on-going support, help and guidance. You are free to contact me at any time with questions about Reiki or for help, support or guidance.

Here are ways I can help you:

Individual Healing Sessions
Reiki Training
Professional Development for Reiki Practitioners
Research and Development of Institutional Reiki Programs.

Thank you!

We believe that the best way to heal is by helping others to heal themselves. Reiki is a wonderful technique that carries a great gift – the gift of being aware of what you already have inside...
Our wish is to bring people back to themselves, and to keep remembering that the Divine is within all of us, always.

Please call or Email with any questions!

With Love & Light,

M. & E. Moghazy

| ezmi@gmx.com |

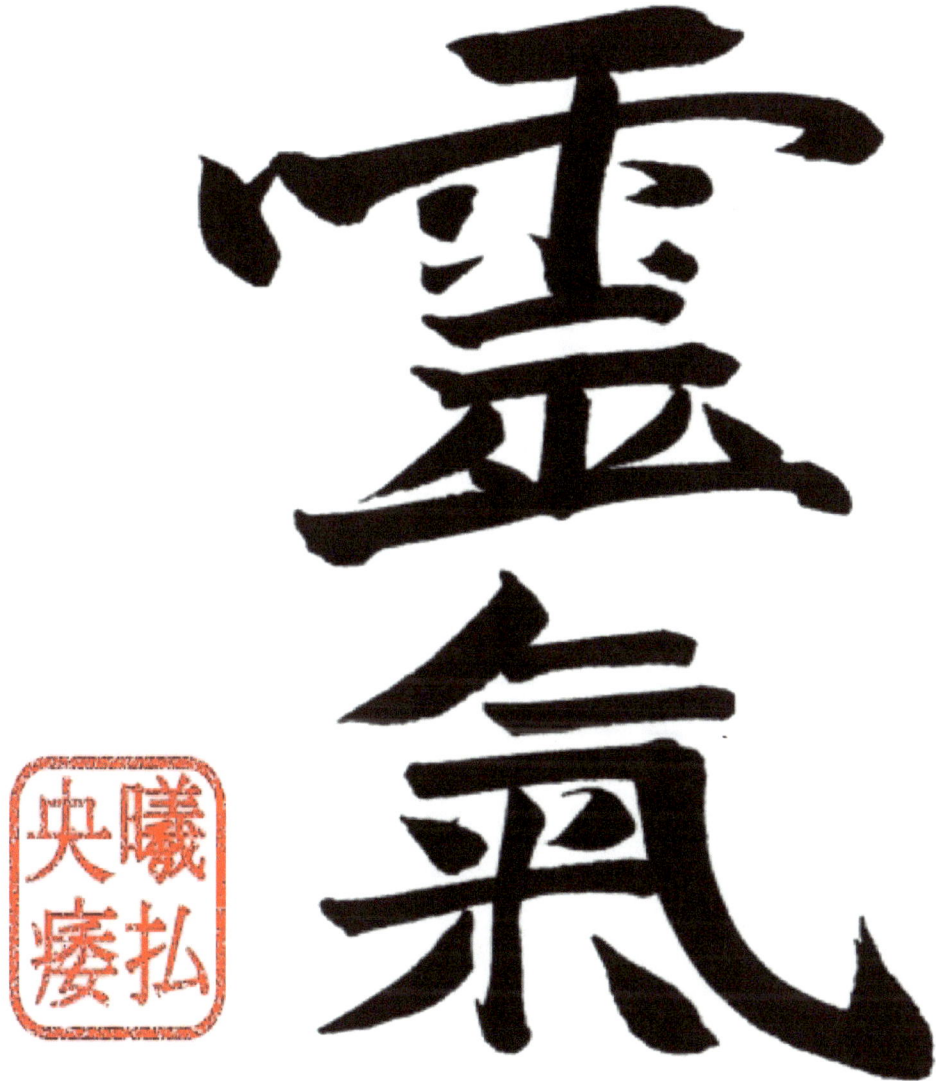